Live Your Health

LIVE YOUR HEALTH

by

**Reuben Halpern
& Joshua Halpern**

ROSS BOOKS

P.O.BOX 4340
BERKELEY, CALIF.
94704

To Berry, Evelyn, Harvey, Joshua, and Betty B. for incalculable gifts
. . . and to all those who listened during the gestation.   — Reuben

To my mother, father, my dear friends whom I cherish, and my beloved
sister Toby.   — Joshua

Halpern, Reuben
    Live Your Health.

    1. Holistic medicine. 2. Mental health 3. Health. 4. Emotions.
5. Self. 6. Nutrition.
I. Halpern, Joshua, joint author. II. Title.
RA790.5.H25   613   79-22622
ISBN 0;89496;020-2

ROSS BOOKS
P.O.BOX 4340
BERKELEY, CALIF.
94704

Foreword

The Paths Of Change

You have seen their faces: the happy people! You don't see too many but you remember them. Especially their eyes. Their eyes drink up life and expect more. They are on the crest of life. It's as if they are riding a wave — while having time to look around too. You say of such people: they "have it together".

You particularly see those faces in children who still have "it" together before the forces of their environment break "it" down and install fear, anxiety, and disease.

And so if you look around at the world you see nations, classes, races, sexes, generations in conflict. Fragmentation. Usually war — sometimes cold, sometimes hot. Poverty, unemployment, disease, malaise. But why go on? You know the story as well as we do.

You see human beings cut off, alienated, from the society they live in, the people they associate with, the work they do, and the products they make. It seems to most that they are not in charge of their world, that they are victims of incalculable and uncontrollable forces. They receive global double messages telling them that they are precious but dispensable, capable but superfluous, richly endowed but lowly. Is it any wonder that the endemic sicknesses of our world are cancer and schizophrenia? Why must these things be?

Check out the faces of your neighbors or your friends or your fellow townspeople — or the members of your family. They too are apt to look drawn, worried, disturbed. They seem to operate on automatic pilot even when the sun is shining bright, even when they're surrounded by people who love them. Why don't they reach out and touch?

Think of the people you know well. Think of their bodies. Aren't most out of shape? Out of energy? Very likely they don't walk straight and proud. Why aren't their eyes bright and alert like a child's? What has happened?

Their spirit, their attitude toward life — isn't that apt to be depressed? (Try to remember how children look when they go out to play!) What has happened to the faith they used to manifest? Why do they just plod on and on when they know — even though they can't feel — that the sun does shine, that people can love and work together, that health — total health — can be won? Why have they lost heart?

We don't know the full answer, of course — just bits and pieces. But perhaps a few key ones we do know that might guide you on a new path that could lead to much more satisfaction.

Obviously, political changes have to take place to open up possibilities for more widespread individual growth. But, on the other hand, many crucial discoveries applicable by individuals have been made; and after all it is *individuals* who make the politics that changes the world. Moreover, when you change the world you change yourself. So the ways of change are interwoven and either way we win.

Perhaps better than "discoveries" we should say we have put some things *together* that clarify and integrate the living process so we can change. Some, perhaps, you are already familiar with and yet are wondering: *How does it all fit together?*

Together, oneness — those are the key words in our vocabulary. It's what healing means: making it whole, one, getting it together. Healing starts with the whole organism, with the body and the psyche, with the way they flow together; and it is here, at this point, where we shall be working. But we warn, predict, and hope that healing cannot proceed far unless personal relationships are dealt with, for we are not islands; in fact relationships form a global network connecting family, lovers, friends, associates, acquaintances to peoples at the very ends of the planet — since we are all one.

Actually the making of *this book* has been a "wholing process" involving a father and son who had separated in the early years of their relationship but then confronted the wall that divided them and battered it down to reach out and meet anew.

So that for us this is more than a book: it is also a "togethering," a collaboration of two generations, for its writing has required the encounter of two human realities with differing world views who made a decision to work together in order to aid others in the healing process. Our very writing has become proof of the process it advocates — the process of healing, or wholing, of oneness.

We have written for those especially who are also on a path of change that can lead to a combining, a re-uniting, of body and psyche, of food and flesh, being and feeling, dreaming and acting, and doing and believing — and ultimately, we do believe, of nations and peoples.

We see holistic healing as a world view in which our lives are experienced as totally connected with the biological, psychological, and spiritual parts of our nature as well as with all the beings on the planet and the life force in everything. It is a view in accord with modern physics and the new parapsychology as well as with the ancient cultures of the East and the intuitive knowings of all indigenous peoples.

We sense that you and millions of others like us know deep inside that it is time to change and that it is time to give up the roles you have been conditioned to play so that we can all fulfill our true natures.

Healing is simply a way of giving form, direction, and meaning to this search; for we know that it can be lonely, and some falter and don't pursue it to new ways of living — and *that* after all is the goal, the living it.

Healing can be painful. Often a "crisis" precedes the healing — in fact promotes it. Struggle is necessary for all change, but you will persevere if you remember the goal: the convergence of your physical, psychological and spiritual natures into their essential oneness.

One further comment: Reuben has contributed most of the material on mental aspects of the path — and Joshua, the biological and ecological aspects. But so frequently have we ignored these artificial boundaries that we can only say finally — *We* did it!

We hope you profit from the doing.

Reuben Halpern
Joshua Halpern

Table Of Contents

THE WORLD OF FEELING

Feelings are meant to be felt, but not *necessarily* followed.

The Starting Point:

WHO ARE WE?

Who are we — we humans? We call ourselves "women," "men," but who are we? What are we about? What is our potential? Are we selfish? loving? good? evil? all of these? What do they mean? It seems the quest for oneness begins in divisions. Must it?

Mark Twain bitterly said: "All that I care to know is that a man* is a human being — that is enough for me; he can't be any worse".

More than ten centuries before Twain, Sophocles rhapsodized: "There are many wonderful things in nature, but the most wonderful of all is man *".

In between these two polar points of view an infinite variety of opinions, diatribes, and paeans have been expressed about us — us humans. Why is that? Why the confusion? Is there a way out? Is there a bridge that crosses over to a new confluence — to a joining of these clashing waters?

Or is there a starting point before the conflict begins that perhaps our children — or theirs — can look forward to?

In both cases we think the answer is Yes, but we must take a brief journey to find that Yes — a journey that begins with the Self.

Within the Self there are no divisions. Within the Self there is an island of calm — haven't you felt it? Within the Self there is a knowing that all is well — haven't you sensed it? We believe that within the Self we know that we are loving, creative, intelligent, and joyous — haven't you experienced it?

We do not believe that all our experiences in the "real world" can fully submerge these vital knowings. Obviously we cannot prove we're right. We can only experience these knowings as, we are sure, you have also. But there are some clues to our true nature even in the "real" world. You can find them in unhurt

---

*Please think "woman" too.

children — if you catch them young enough. Recall now (if there are no young children in your life): How their eyes shine! How curious and intelligent they are! How truly artistic, how honest, how loving, how delightfully various! How unique!

And there are clues in our adult selves too. We'd like to help you find them. They are not far away. They are as close as you are...Let's take a short trip together now to find the bridge that we all seek.

All you need is a favorite chair, a quiet light, perhaps some music that fosters repose, and your desire to explore .

THE BRIDGE

Close your eyes now and get rid of all the old air in your lungs. Do this three or four times, each time unhurriedly allowing fresh air to return. Now follow your breath for three to five minutes: that is, just watch it; as it comes in, mentally say *in* and when it goes out, say *out*. Just that. (It is amazing how we free our Self to observe our true nature through this simple technique.)

Now review your life chronologically for SPECIFIC moments when "somehow" everything you did was right. (Re-discover also how you were feeling at these times.) For example, when were you:

1. Creative?
2. Loving?
3. Courageous?
4. Confident?
5. Productive?

Take your time with this recovery of precious experiences, for they could alter your view of your Self; they could finally be the basis for a new self-image. If feelings well up, allow them to flow — *that* is the healing process. In fact, if possible ask a friend, lover, mate, spouse to review *their* moments at the same time, so that you can come together to share your findings; for feelings can be felt more securely if they are shared. Yet individually this experience can be equally rewarding, so try it! (If you can get a partner, take equal turns listening and sharing.)

Let a day go by before you do this next part so that you will be deeply aware of what you have found. Now with your partner — if you have one — do the breathing described and then look back at SPECIFIC moments when somehow everything you did was wrong. (Once again re-discover how you were feeling at these times.)

When were you:
1. Unaware?
2. Unhelpful?
3. Scared?
4. Unconfident?
5. Unproductive?

Once again, take your time in this retrospective search. Be hospitable to your feelings. Feelings are neither good nor bad: they are simply to be felt at appropriate times.

We couldn't even guess what you recovered in these two reviews because we are all unique; but in your uniqueness you share a commonality with all humans — so that we venture to say that when things went right and you were truly "ON" you were also feeling good . . .and when things went wrong, you were feeling bad.

We are also sure that feeling good means feeling good about yourself, just as feeling bad means feeling bad about yourself — it's just that simple. (Feeling good and bad, of course, have nothing to do with avoiding or being deluged with misfortune, hardship, or struggle. On the contrary. We can feel very good while struggling!)

Furthermore, we believe: you have never hurt anyone when you have truly loved yourself. And yet we are not misty-eyed dreamers. You have hurt people, and so have we. We're aware of the "real world": its cruelty, its wars, the murders, the plunder; the vast injustices, the barbarous inequalities; the grievous stupidities based on distinctions of sex, race, and nationality; the forced labor camps, the "detention" centers, the concentration camps with their factory-like precision...

Where is the bridge then? Where is the opening to our essential positive nature that we claim to be "truly human"?

First we must look for where the waters divide before we can build the bridge. They divide when we feel bad about ourselves — we have ascertained that. Now: where does self-invalidation come from? What is its source?

We have to start in the real world — a world that, if we look at it objectively, we must admit is a "power world"; that is, it permits those in power to profit economically, politically, psychologically, and spiritually through the domination of others.

This is not only personal domination. It's also a *system of power* that utilizes the hierarchies of class, race, age, nationality (and so many more subtle categories) so that all of us — even those in power — have our place and role in order to manipulate and be mainpulated *predictably*.

Of course systems of power are based on *personal* domination, which can only prevail if human beings surrender part of their power, part of their belief in themselves. This is easy to observe in the "lower" class, the "weaker" sex, the minorities — the obviously manipulated and oppressed. Not only do they accede to actual displays of real power ("majority rule," tradition, ideology, the police, etc.) but, more importantly, they *incorporate* the "necessary" beliefs — really rationalizations — that justify their oppression: they *recreate* themselves to become less intelligent, less resourceful, less creative, less fully endowed than the leaders and rulers of the society.

Incorporation means to believe these rationalizations *within the body* — to believe them unthinkingly, instantaneously. This "demands" self-addressed prejudice, self-inflicted invalidation, self-directed denigration. The oppressed must cooperate in their oppression! Few oppressed people believe in their full humanity. If many did, they would have it! (If you are oppressed or if you know someone who is, reflect on the validity of this analysis.)

What is not so clear is that the wielders of power must also surrender part of their humanity; for as manipulators they must also be manipulated by the power system. In order to rule they must *desensitize* themselves to the humanity of all people, to the beauty of all people, to the possibilities in all people — or else they could not function. Desensitization means not only blindness to others but to themselves also: it is both an emotional and spiritual occlusion.

On the level of sociology the power system is very subtle; but on our level of human healing it is very simple, and the simplicity is that this vast and complicated system of power could not last one day longer if its victims (all of us) felt good about ourselves.

In other words, self-invalidation is the psychological keystone of this vast system of human engineering that we call the real world.

We're getting closer to the bridge, but we're not there yet. We have discovered the source; but now we need to find out how the source works its "wondrous ways" to produce such willing subjects.

Once again this is a vast simplicity, but it is essentially true: our home, our parents (or those that function in that role) are the initial primary indoctrinating agents in that extensive assembly line that ultimately produces the "willing" victim. (Obviously the schools, the media, and the immediate environment reinforce all that we originally learn.)

Why do they do it? Why do those that love us get us ready to serve the power system? They would say: *because* they love us! Because they are afraid we will suffer if we are not indoctrinated. They are afraid that if we expose our full humanity in the cultural marketplace we will be destroyed; so they prepare us to devalue ourselves before we are devalued by the world.

But this too is very subtle, for it is basically not a conscious process. Few parents would consciously deprive their children of their birthright. But parents were also children, and *they* were deprived: they were put down, they were invalidated, *they were made ready for the system*. And that experience of psychic *make-ready* becomes the (largely unconscious) behavioral model for their children.

Furthermore psychic make-ready means pain and hurt — the *implantation* of unconscious pain mechanisms (that create rigid behavior patterns) within the child that will insist on replaying like recordings. Furthermore these will replay in that child's children if the pain is passed on to them.

Make-ready is an easy term for the hard ways of invalidation, for all the hurt and pain that humans must feel — for being less than human. It also includes the *substitute behavior* that is "installed" in young children through unconscious pain mechanisms which dictate the way we're "supposed to" behave. It is also a term for the way we "have to" behave once we have incorporated the pain. If we "have to" behave in a prescribed way once a "button" is pushed, then we cannot react to the world in a rational fashion; we foreclose on our most precious possession, our power to reason, which can suit the solution to the unique moment.

Make-ready also includes the patterns of behavior that both anesthetize the pain and correlate all the recordings so that eventually they can seem logical and even reasonable.

For now let us say that this is how psychological continuity through the generations is maintained, but we shall have much more to say about pain mechanisms later on. This is no tale about dread human fate, however, for change is just as integral to human history as continuity.

If you have any doubts, study the clild-rearing practices of previous generations. Only within the last two-hundred years have parents stopped killing their unwanted female children. The need of human beings to be and to grow and to change the world — thereby changing themselves — continually asserts and re-asserts itself throughout history. We particularly are interested in producing change, in rewriting personal scenarios.

But first it would be wise to examine our sense of ourselves, which is often decisively determined by those pain-induced behavior patterns which then become the foundation of our presumed "characters."It's an insidious process indeed. First we are hurt. We then defend ourselves against further hurt with protective psychic structures; finally these structures are pinned on us as our "characters"!

That is why it is absolutely necessary to examine our self-image in order to lay the ghosts of the past so that we can determine who we really are. Frankly, we are not sure of what "character" means. We do know it generally describes *imposed* behavior and therefore spells dangerous assumptions about the individual. All in all it is a perilous concept.

We also know that people are unique and therefore have *inner* characters; but these are so camouflaged by outer labels and installed patterns that until we can come home to our loving, creative, intelligent, and zestful natures, the labels will be straightjackets rather than enhancing attire.

Perhaps with the following simple exercise we can begin to lay the ghosts .

THE SCENARIO

Let's first find out "your" labels. Below are 20 characterological pairs. Ask yourself, "Which one of the pair do I identify with?" Write it down (We'll use this information shortly.) Please remember this is not a test. It is simply a step in uncovering the labeling process.

1.	happy	1.	sad
2.	friendly	2.	reserved
3.	optimistic	3.	pessimistic
4.	resilient	4.	rigid
5.	zestful	5.	gloomy
6.	open	6.	secretive
7.	outgoing	7.	retiring
8.	trusting	8.	suspicious
9.	cooperative	9.	individualistic
10.	loving	10.	selfish
11.	confident	11.	unsure
12.	ambitious	12.	lazy
13.	assertive	13.	passive
14.	courageous	14.	fearful
15.	determined	15.	wishy-washy
16.	curious	16.	indifferent
17.	intelligent	17.	stupid
18.	resourceful	18.	limited
19.	creative	19.	imitative
20.	self-supporting	20.	dependent

Now repeat the breathing routine described on Page 14 for THE BRIDGE. Take your time. You can also do this alone or with a friend. The exercise should be broken up into four 90-minute sessions corresponding with the four groups of attributes. If you identify rather consistently with the positives in the left-hand column, take just as much time. Enjoy your good fortune!

We must also repeat: your potential is all the positives in the left-hand column. They are your birthright, literally! You will only get full value from this work if you believe this. For now at least *be receptive to the possibility*.

Start with the first pair (happy-sad). Which one do you identify with?

If it is with the positive (happy), celebrate! RIGHT NOW recapture for your friend and/or yourself the memorably happy times you have experienced. Once again: take your time (this is important).

If it is with the negative - when? where? how? and with whom? was this label first fixed. What made you feel there was no alternative? Further: How has the label affected your life? (If you have feelings, let them happen. SHOUT! SCREAM! CRY! SHAKE! Hit a pillow. Have a tantrum. IT'S O.K.!) How many repetitions of the initial imprinting do you vividly recall? Recapture them now.

Do as many pairs as you have time for within the 90-minute period. Save the rest for another session. This work is important and deserves your best energy.

REWRITING THE SCENARIO

Now you can do something about those negatives you have thought to be you but actually are only ALIEN attitudes, perceptions, standards, ways of feeeling and being that were foisted on you when you had to adopt them to survive. NOW you have a choice!

Decide that you are going to give energy and attention to your true identity, to that irreduceable you that still hungers for sun and space.

1.   Begin with the first group of positive qualities. Look at them. Truly relive RIGHT NOW times in your life when you were not a slave to alien tapes. Recapture these experiences. What kind of day was it? Whom were you with? How did the sun and the ground you walked on and the body that was YOUR instrument feel? What was unique about the precious moment?

2.   Close your eyes and breathe deeply of your essence, nourishing it with each breath. Each breath can be a silent vow to continually nourish your RESURGENT self. If the pain of those "wasted" years seems too heavy and tears form, let them flow. (Please remember they were not wasted: you truly did the best you could and could not have arrived at this point one second sooner. Truly!)

3.   Continue to sustain your retrieved identity. Close your eyes and direct fresh energy to your stirring Self. With eyes still closed adopt a stance, a facial expression, a way of being in the world that captures the retrieved identity you have rescued for your present life.

4.   NOW open your eyes and hold on to your repossessed identity. Maintain the posture and expression for four minutes. (We recommend that you do this three times a day until you feel YOU!)

5.   Choose an activity — whether work or play — in which your new self can be itself: It could be dancing or art or a new hobby or a volunteer job. Make a commitment to do it as often as possible. It may mean a new vocation or a new friend.

The full story about feeling good and feeling bad has still to be pursued. Renewing and reorienting as the above exercise can be, we still have to answer the question, HOW is it that we feel bad, that we do feel invalidation? What happens? How do the waters divide?

They divide in the process we call hurt or pain. It *is* a process. It is a process that affects the whole organism: the body, the mind... (How inadequate our vocabulary is for describing what we are — for it so divides us! Nevertheless — if we treat ourselves as one, if we do not listen to the siren songs of those in the medical and psychiatric professions who see the mind and the body as two entities, we can bridge the waters. The new vocabulary will eventually happen...)

We do not know physiologically what takes place when hurt occurs; we only know operationally, and so do you.

Our thinking abilities collapse. (It feels as if they shut down.) We become "scared out of our wits"; "numbed with grief"; "crazy with rage"; "out of our head" with pain — so that the quintessence of the human being, our ability to think and act creatively in each and every unqiue situation, vanishes.

And yet the self does not cease to operate. Our senses still record and photograph. We still feel and see. But the data pouring in become skewed. The "facts" are distorted and therefore misinterpreted. The mind's sorting operations that group similar data together so that they can be recalled efficiently jumble and misshuffle them instead. Each time we are hurt this process repeats itself; and yet we must make decisions with these data reagardless, for life must go on. And so we repetitively draw on these past hurt experiences (with their distorted data and conclusions) whenever a new experience occurs that we associate with them.

Thus we remain prisoners of the past rather than architects of the future. We re-act instead of act. When one realizes how often we are hurt in any single day, the effects could be staggering... And yet with all the hurt, with all the rigid "solutions" to ever-new challenges, human beings survive, prosper, and progress. How do we do it?

Have you ever seen a child who gets hurt? She stubs her toe or hits her head on a chair, let us say. What does she do? The child begins to cry of course. (She will cry harder if someone pays attention to her; if someone touches her or holds her she might even bawl.) The extent of crying will depend on the intensity of hurt, but we know that eventually the child will suddenly stop crying, look around as if the world were full of myriad possibilities, and be on her way — happy as the proverbial lark. What has happened?

Again we don't know physiologically but we do know operationally. We know that the hurt has been somehow erased and the data therefore that came in skewed by virtue of it are now un-skewed so that the child is free to grow again unreactively. Somehow the crying healed the pain. (Most people erroneously believe that the crying *is* the pain!) Now the feeling of pain is gone (not the memory of the incident, which is probably clearer than ever before.). We might also point out that if this crying did not take place, the pain would be *embodied* as long as that individual lived: pain retention has been ascertained thousands of times...

The body in its wisdom has different circuitries for healing different pains: For grief, tears, sobbing; for heavy fear, trembling and cold perspiration; light fear, laughter and cold perspiration; for heavy anger, "furious" noises and movement with warm perspiration; for light anger, laughter and warm perspiration; boredom (probably the most painful of all emotions!), animated — though often preceded by reluctant — talking.

For want of a better term we call the *triggers* (tears, laughter, shaking, etc.) that set off the healing process *discharge*. (All in all it's not a bad term though it does have unfortunate connotations.) It *does* seem like discharge when you've experienced it: first there is that heavy emotional and physical atmosphere of hurt in which we must exist; and then proof! magically it is gone — as if discharged, as if lightning had cleared our atmosphere.

Discharge is feeling the hurt — not talking about it or analyz-ing it. It is not acting crazy or outlandish or destructively "angry" (these behaviors we call "acting out"; they are actually ways of avoiding discharge). Discharge is a letting go in order to feel.

And the result? New clarity. A new reorientation. New think-ing, new perceptions, new decisions, new approaches, new growth. New growth that is based on an accurate assessment of sense data rather than on a reactive muddled formula. So that the result of feeling is rationality — a wedding of productive thinking with congruent feelings. And rationality is the prime achievement of the human species.

Children, of course, are the great authorities on discharge, but we are all capable of it though we suppress it, while somewhere we know deep down that we need it. Ask yourself...

What has happened to inhibit this lifesaving gift? How can we rebuild the bridge?

The clue to the first question is the male's comparative inability to discharge. He plays it "cool" and "tough". No sissy he. He responds to an inner signal for discharge as to an enemy interrogator. He is a MAN and will not bend unless broken! He plays his cards close to his chest and they will be revealed only if wrested from him.

And yet we know that male babies cry just like the female ones. Therefore we must look to the culture for an answer, and so we discover a clue: In almost all cultures we find that men are almost the exclusive wielders of power. (We are not talking about domination, which is personal, but power, which is social and political. Women often dominate, they rarely have power.)

Now one thing is clear about the roles of men in power relationships: they cannot be themselves. If they are, they will be defeated. It is dangerous to reveal yourself if you are the victim; and it is foolish if you are in charge.

There was also a primitive justification for the supression of male discharge that was operative in the hunting stage of society but probably still persists. Discharge then could have been not only foolish but fatal. A display of hurt or a gasp of fear could have made one vulnerable to an immediate charge by a hostile animal.

No wonder men look at discharge as weakening . . .as unmanly. No wonder they insure that their sons too learn the message at least by the time they are adolescents. And no wonder men rarely discharge even within the bosom of their families, for patterns of behavior become unconscious; and no matter how lowly outside the home, they wield power within it. Ravaged by diseases caused by tensions that discharge can release, no wonder men die 10-15 years earlier than the "weaker" sex.

On the other hand the family structure, in which women have traditionally operated, has been determined by *external* power relationships over which they've had no control — so that their priority has always been the basic needs of human beings, particularly the children's, within the family.

Comparatively, therefore, women discharge more freely than men. But they can never be truly themselves either in a society based on power relationships that limit their freedom not only outside the family but within its male-dominated structure.

Obviously men and women together need to work out ways of both sharing and releasing their feelings so that the power structures themselves will eventually be replaced by the primacy of human needs.

Otherwise, men and women will do what they have always done to "relieve" the pressure and tension of suppressed hurts — they will live *symbolically*.

That is, rather than satisfying their *true needs*, they will spend an inordinate amount of energy in not only suppressing them but in substituting self-destructive symbolic needs for them — so that their true feelings will not surface.

Withdrawn and depressive behavior will thus "replace" fear and grief; eating and chattering will "replace" love; daily rigid routines will "replace" despair; cynicism and "realism" will "replace" joy and excitement; incessant activity, inner boredom; and status symbols, a positive self-image. The list, of course, is endless...

Nor is this the end of the endlessness, for the body too will "cooperate" in a multitude of symbolic distortions, rigidities, tics, aches, spasticities, dysfunctions, lesions, breakdowns, and finally the overarching symbol — death.

The purpose of this book therefore is to foster the return to our selves — to our needs, to our feelings, so that we can eat when we're hungry, love when we're caring, cry when we're hurting, and rejoice when we're happy.

A Friend Is At Hand:

THE ART OF SELF-COUNSELING

What do you do when you're hurting — and alone? When you can almost feel the tears (or the fear, or anger) and there's no friend to talk to? When you want to *release* the feelings, get rid of them, *discharge* them — instead of suppressing them with food or drink or "will power" and simply accepting this new hurt as your lot in life and thus going a little more dead, a little further away from the vibrant person you really are?

We say: You do have a friend at hand — your left hand! What I am about to tell you is based on scientific knowledge of human psychology. Our bodies tend to operate with their right side as controller, the willer, the doer. It is the servant of what most psychologists call the ego (our "personality", our persona).

The left side of our bodies is a moderating force. It intuits, imagines, feels, dreams. It somehow *is*! The left hand is the dreamer . . .

(Inspect your own left and right sides. They will probably differ subtly but amazingly. It is most evident in the eyes. The right tends to be fearful, calculating, darting, mercurial; but the left — soft, accepting, aware. As we become more centered, more "grounded", these differences will tend to balance out, however.)*

Your left hand is also the counselor. Let's say you are upset. First, calm yourself with the breathing exercise described on page 14. Now allow your left hand to firmly — but kindly — take charge of your being.

Have the left hand take hold of the right. Let it soothe the whole arm. Let it be a strong - but supportive - parent; for that's what you need. Let the left hand do what it intuitively knows you need it

---

* It is important to note that these differences correlate with right-handedness. Left-handed people have different "geographies."

to do. Let it stroke and soothe and calm and rest where it knows you need it to. Give it the opportunity to be free. Don't stop it. It will amaze you sometimes with its audacious knowing.

Now tell it your story. Tell it what's troubling you. Allow it to be in charge, it is your counselor. It can help even under surprising conditions. For example, I was disturbed a few days before writing this. I soon had to drive to work to help others; but I needed help myself, I had feelings that needed expression. And there was no one to talk to — but me.

So me it was soon after I got into the car. (I can do this quite safely while driving!) My "counselor" initiated the session:

Left Hand: What are you feeling, Reuben?

Reuben: I feel that I'm just mucking around in distress that's preventing me from truly realizing myself. I know that I'm on a high plateau and that I've traveled a long way to get here; but I'm feeling the plateau, I'm feeling the *stuckness* rather than all the barriers I've broken, all the blocks I've smashed, all the feelings I've worked through. I'm not happy with myself. (considerable anger, frustration)

Left Hand: Reuben, what have you done in the last several years that you are proud of? Tell me about them — and tell me about them proudly, with proud voice, proud body, proud smile. Sit up!

Reuben: (Feeling very angry.) I'm tired of this! Leave me alone! I want to be *there* already! I'm tired of flailing around in the surf. It's about time I arrived! (An unwilling smile breaks through.)

Left Hand: Reuben, get to work...

Reuben: O.K. What do you want to know?

Left Hand: (gently) Come on, tell me what you've done.

Reuben: (reluctantly) I don't know where it started, maybe right after I was born (bitter laughter); but I guess I'll start with Fritz[1] and Esalen[2] and Big Sur during the Sixties, when my heart used to sing with the beauty of the sun and the air and the sea and my vision of a beautiful life liberated from fear and longing and hurt. It was so beautiful! (tears)

Left Hand: Say that again.

Reuben: It was so beautiful. (tears) I was so beautiful! (laughter, tears)

Left Hand: What are you thinking?

Reuben: It was so frightening. I was so scared! The fear of exposure paralyzed me, and yet I wanted to move. I did move — perhaps as much from listening to the struggles of others as from having the spotlight shine on me. Those were good days. (tears) They were days of hope. (tears) I used to "fly" from those workshops past the arching bridges and high cliffs of the Sur to the white sands of Carmel and Monterey back to Berkeley, buoyed up for days.

Left Hand: What are you thinking?

Reuben: I felt I was on my way. I *was* on my way! (tears)

Left Hand: Say that again.

Reuben: I was on my way. (tears) (I then recounted other chapters on my journey that were painful, liberating and joyous: the many self-explorations that highlighted my training and apprenticeship in psychotherapy.) I've been on my way so many times and for so long. When will it end?

Left Hand: When will it end, Reuben?

Reuben: Never.

Left Hand: Yeah . . . How does that grab you?

Reuben: It feels O.K. now that I can see clearly the line between me and my distresses; but sometimes when they take over, it's hard.

---

[1] Frederick S. Perls, M.D., the founder of Gestalt Therapy and the presiding genius of Esalen during the latter part of his life.

[2] Esalen Institute is the famous growth center in Big Sur, California, where so many of the innovative ideas of humanistic psychology were first tried out.

Left Hand: Then what do you do?
Reuben: Find a friend — or you.
Left Hand: Yeah. I love you, Reuben. Don't forget that.
Reuben: I never do — for long, (laughter)

The above session was real. It took place, it is not a synthetic production. In fact, it was difficult to recreate even a portion of the excitement it generated. For one thing, it had to be vastly shortened; but even that doesn't explain the loss of magic. Perhaps all we can say is: writing *about* something is not experiencing it. But it's the best we can do.

And yet although it felt very special indeed, it was an "ordinary" session — I've had dozens similar, many of much deeper import. So the question is, how do you go about it? how do they happen?

They happen through trust, through love. And isn't it true that often the greatest love a friend or counselor can give is to listen? — to listen with no hidden agendas, with respect, with deep appreciation for the life that is unfolding.

Your right side might have advice to give, criticism to make, judgments to deliver, even scores to settle. Forget them, swallow them. They are not helpful. All of us keep up a running battle with ourselves - judging ourselves to death - but we don't need it and we *need not to get it* once we understand and appreciate our unique ability to switch hands, to declare a truce, and to listen with love. If you do nothing else but listen, you will have given yourself a great gift. (What do you think people pay expensive psychiatrists for? P.S. You might become a better listener!)

The next question is, What to listen for? The answer is: focus, energy, excitement. If your "client" takes the bit in his/her teeth and begins running with it, then don't interrupt. Let it happen. But if you see that the subject has suddenly shifted and/or that the energy level has fallen, bring your client back to the original focus. Don't allow avoidance. Listen!

For instance, your counselor might say: Looks like you've stopped dealing with all the hurt around ——————. How about getting back to it? You might then reply, "Well, if you insist".(If you are resisting strongly, your counselor had *better* insist!).

Especially if a statement has brought tears or anger or fear in its wake, gently insist that your client return to it.

Whatever the strong feeling, ask for the statement to be repeated; "milk" it until the feeling no longer discharges. Then ask "What are you thinking?" to discover connective feelings, thoughts, or situations that need to be investigated and milked. Be a hawk! Follow every scent. It is amazing how objective you can become. (After all, who knows you best?)

If anger erupts, then invite your client to shout or scream or hit a pillow or have a tantrum or say "grrr" or whatever is appropriate. (Again — you ought to know what *is* appropriate.) Just remember one thing about anger — in most cases it is a "cover feeling" for deeper emotions — usually hurt and sorrow, often fear. So don't be surprised by the tears: most clients are reluctant to admit to loss or hurt. Anger is one of the few validated feelings in our culture, so it is marvelous (unaware) camouflage — especially for males.

Fear is most difficult to deal with in self-counseling. It needs very close support — very likely from another — especially if it is deep. The best way to handle fear in any case is to treat it lightly. Make a joke of it (even though it's not funny) so that you will be able to release some of the tension around its edges — to "bleed" it, as it were. Laughter is the supreme antidote to fear. Tension helps to keep fear in check; when it slackens therefore, deeper fears can surface, and perhaps shaking and sweating might ensue.

But don't count on it. It is extraordinarily helpful just to release the tension. Then you will begin to *feel* the fear instead of suppressing it and embodying it — thus creating all sorts of psychosomatic illnesses as a result. It is important to remember that fear is a useful, lifesaving emotion that becomes deadly only when we suppress it. We needn't fear it!

Fear actually becomes an ally when we don't fear it. Encourage your client to kid around. If he's about to apply for a new job or ask for a raise in pay, have him say: "Everyone wants me to advance!" or perhaps, "I'm so confident I astound myself!" Then watch the laughter melt the fear.

A slightly deeper level of fear can be contacted by asking your client to say something cockily scary and then roll the shoulders while saying "brrr." (Very likely prickles of fear will then race up and down the spine.)

Once again, the main strategy is lightness. Fear can sink a person more quickly than a hearse; and when you're sunk, nothing works.

The deeper discharge of fear through shaking and cold and/or hot sweating should not be expected in self-counseling. Extremely threatening feelings will require a professional counselor or a good friend who can give you the support you need while you discharge your way out of the dark tunnel. (Ask to be held tight while you shake — this works wonders —; after all you probably wouldn't have been scared in the first place if you hadn't been alone!).

The main thing for your counselor to beware of is self-invalidation. (If we didn't do this to ourselves we wouldn't need counseling in the first place!). We are all expert at this because *we* know where it hurts. But this self-wounding knowledge can be turned to advantage by the counselor if he/she can revolve the put-down 360 degrees in order to discharge the hurt. For example:

Client: I'm a failure. I really botched it. There's a demon in me that screws up everything I want to do right.

Counselor: How about saying — proudly — "I'm a great success!"Don't say it glibly. Think first about the fight you always put up to meet the challenge. Think how hard it's been — and feel it. Think about the successes — even though partial — you have achieved and then say it, *proudly*.

Client: It's true! I have tried! And it hasn't been easy! I have come a long way! I have done_____. And I've also done ——————————. And what about ————————! That was damned hard! I've really done the best I could! (Very likely tears and laughter will vie for expression at this point...)

Counselor: Of course you have. So how about saying it now — proudly!

Client: I'm a great success...(More feelngs, animated talking, and perhaps insight could also ensue.)

Who knows how such a session would turn out for you? Perhaps after recounting your successes — and deriving the strength that accrues from self-realization — you would recall those in your life who put you down. (You can be certain that if you put yourself down there was a prior figure who showed you how!)

Then your counselor could ask you to talk to these figures with the strength and awareness you have right now in order to redress your righteous grievances.   Or else your counselor could simply ask you to stick to saying, "I'm a great success," as you cull and deal with counter-feelings and counter-thoughts that will be dislodged by this tremendous statement.

It *is* a tremendous statement — although it might *feel* simplistic and even downright fatuous — because it is literally true that you have always done the best you could and your best therefore *was* a success. When you really think about that, when you really grasp the profundity of knowing that you could not have done any better in your life, you will begin to move with giant strides; for this profound idea is the taproot of self-acceptance, just as self-acceptance is the activator of change.

Of course there is no formula for a successful self-counseling session. How could there be? We are all different, unique. Yet there are some guidelines. The main one is to be supportive and nurturing — yet not appeasing or coddling. You'll know the difference: if you come out of a session positive, self-affirmative, and with a special definite achievable goal in mind — then you'll know you're on the right track.

Actually, the danger is not in self-appeasement but in self-abasement. Stop putting yourself down — in session or out. We don't need character assassins. We need friends who can listen to our hurts, angers, and fears so that we can get off dead center and move into the world more rational, more loving, more creative — always closer to the marvelous humans we really are.

Don't let your session become an exercise in self-analysis. This too generally culminates in put-down and let-down. Why-questions are the main weapons of analysis — avoid them. Why's are interminable and lead to impotence. We don't want dissection but reconstruction. We don't want intellectualization but feeling and *being*. And then change!

Client: I don't know why I can't stop procrastinating. I can't accomplish anything! I guess my father was like that too. I hated him for it — I couldn't rely on him for anything. I don't know why he was like that. His brothers weren't, and *my* brother isn't like that either — he gets out and does things. I guess he identified with my mother — I don't know why. I don't know, I just don't.

Counselor: This doesn't seem to be getting you anywhere but in a funk. *How* do you procrastinate? *What* do you do? Maybe we can change your script ...Let's work on *that!*

We're not opposed to intellect, to *real* thinking — only to intellectualization, which is mental masturbation in a vacuum. Humans *naturally* think, are *naturally* creative so that when they stop being creative and thoughtful and forward-moving the answer lies in removing the block, which almost invariably is suppressed feelings.* *Feel* your way out of it and you'll be fine — without all the why's to pin you down like a mounted insect. Only *then* will you *think* clearly and productively, for rational behavior *is* the goal. And that *feels* fine!

In other words, your "counselor in residence" need always be alert to your human posibilities? Whenever in doubt, validate, appreciate, love. What better place to start than with yourself?

Now, with your new counseling skills, you can stay on top of not only upsetting distress when a friend or professional counselor is not available but also your *daily* need to deal with regularly recurring feelings of being "down" or sunk. These often surface upon awaking in the morning or getting into bed at night.

There is simply no need to be sunk in the morning until you get your first "hit" of coffee — not that that will be sufficient. Rather, set aside about ten minutes while still in bed for clearing cobwebs caused possibly by disturbing dreams or "down" feelings of being unequal to the imminent day's activities.

---

*Sometimes, of course, lack of information can cause the block.

We shall go in depth into working with unresolved dream material in another chapter; but for now we simply advise recalling the responsible dream with as much detail as possible and then asking yourself how you would like it to have turned out.

Have it turn out that way right then and there! Fantasize the dream you want. You can *change* it. (Fantasies are cut from the same cloth as dreams.) After all, it was *your* dream: you are your dream-maker — producer, director, actor, scene designer, and audience. Get to work — it won't take long — and you will remove the glooms that could cloud your presence most of the morning.

If the morning blahs are caused by feelings of being unequal to the day, then validate yourself — you know how now. Look at your past achievements. They are a precious resource. Cherish them. Don't dismiss them because they are in the past. Really they are not, they are in the *living* present. They can become the sinew of an emergent strong self that knows not only where it's going but where it's been.

Don't *recite* your achievements like a parrot. Your words, tone, facial expression and body should all be — proud! Choose your victories carefully to confront the particular inadequacy you might then be feeling. You know which one will most tellingly knock the underpinnings from a chronic "recording" that has probably been yapping at you for years. Put it in its place with sunlight and laughter and your real worth.

But you are not simply a shopping list of achievements, important though they might be. You are also you: a person with qualities, with goals, with ideals, with beliefs, with a sense of the beautiful and the just, with a capacity to love and create.

Draw on the vast account that is yourself and confront the puny demons that rule only by your abstention. You will soon realize that they will run from your first words of sanity and decision. They cannot stand a postivie point of view. So be cruelly unfair to them with lethal rays of personal power.

At night mental unrest can be caused by the unfinished business of the day: things you didn't do or didn't complete or perhaps didn't do as well as you would have liked to, or maybe didn't do because of fear. It's not easy to fall asleep with agendas like that asking for the floor.

There are two tactics for disposing of unfinished business. The first is to sit up and write out for yourself a list of things to do to set your mind at rest. Put them in chronological order so as to develop a feeling for progression and change. Then be sure to do them so that unfounded worries will *feel* unfounded: you will soon convince yourself that you are reliable and are responsible.

The other tactic is the essential one, the basic one: your unswerving reiteration that you did the best you could. But don't just *say* it — go over the entire action to prove it yourself. That doesn't mean you're perfect — not at all. There are of course things you'd like to change in yourself. What are they? What gets in the way? Can you make plans with a friend or counselor or your own counselor-in-residence to eliminate these blocks by working through the rigid negative feelings that cement them in place. There is a vast difference between having done the best you could and *planning* to do better in the future. Even your negative feelings will soon recognize it and leave the bed — for your rest.

We have spoken about self-counseling as something *to do*, as a way to handle the many psychic problems we must deal with in this highly complex world we live in. There are, of course, also ways of *being* that can be enormously beneficial, and we have allocated a chapter to a central way of being — meditation.

But sometimes it is crucially useful to have a *place* in which to be — your place, a place for your Self, a Safe House. I call mine a study, but that's because I'm a writer and a sometime scholar. The essence of this place is you.

Your "landscape" will be different than mine, the special things that can bring you home to yourself will be different; but the essence will be the same — you. Perhaps it will be a closet or a corner of a room or a garage that you know to be a refuge for affirmation and growth.

Whatever it is, that place will be a part of you and will *trigger* the inner sense of you when you inhabit its space. Begin constructing it in your mind's eye if you have no place like this — and then create it!

It's easy to do. — children do it all the time with a wave of the hand and a blink of the eye and perhaps a doll or a toy train. We all *need* to be "children." (Actually we need to be our own parents giving ourselves permission to be "children".)

In my refuge (this is not a prescription but an example) a drawing of a man has become very important to me. I think of him as Everyman. It is a picture of a person who is gaunt and vulnerable, who has been appalled by horrors, who has seen it all. And yet his body is planted proudly: a force to be reckoned with, a human being for "all that and a' that" (as Bobbie Burns might say.) And when I look at him, I am proud for *my* self. I can even shed a few tears sometimes for my "Brother!"

And there's a poem on the wall that a dear friend wrote about me. It often weakens the cold grip of the past. I must include its last two stanzas:

> Fingertips that speak
> Of love's old
> Hopes
> And destiny's despairs
>
> Silver lad dreaming still
> Beside the river
> Of tomorrow
> With years grown young
> In the alchemy
> Of an autumn dream.

To the right of Everyman are snapshots of my now dead original family and my present beautiful family — and so much else: certificates, licenses, memorabilia. And what do they all mean? — the panorama of a life. The depth of a life. The things that "whole" me, center me. They allow me to see myself in a broad biographical, emotional, and spiritual perspective — so that when somehow my self-image slips I can look at these reminders with shock: "Who-me?" Yes! Me!!

They are a way to oneness, and we are suggesting that you enable yourself to rediscover the dream that is you when you find it hard to remember so that you can soon stand erect again feeling that it *has* been worth the candle. If there are feelings that get in the way of your rediscovery — release them, cry them away, so that you can sail serene in the stream of time. Give yourself that time — in your Place . . .

As Hillel said a long time ago: "If you're not for yourself, who will be?" True, he went on to say: "If you are for yourself alone, who are you?" But that's not another question. It's the same one. For it's our belief that true self-love complements — in fact, guarantees — the love of others.

It *is* all one. Strengthening the Self through self-counseling and other ways can only redound to the benefit of us all.

Servants Or Saboteurs:

THE FUNCTION OF FEELINGS

My wife and I received a frightening letter at the time I started this chapter. It was from a friend: about 55, married and divorced three times, attorney and succcessful writer, a brilliant woman who has gone through "a lot of changes" (as she would say) in the last few years.

She started off with a slight bit of typical chitchat and then got down to "it":

"Here it's been 'dramatic' for interior and exterior reasons both. I had heavy dealings with my parents which climaxed in my mother's suicide. (She then briefly reported where her father is living.) I also had a heavy love affair which took me to some strange places. I have done no legal work but am about to resume my practice. An exciting case has just fallen into my lap.

"Fortunately I have picked myself up from the depths. I know I was right in following my personal thread home to my parents even though it seems I caused a disaster. But feelings are no idle playthings and I followed mine. And I'm better now.

"Sometime in late August will return to Denver."

(She then added a few details about how to reach her and closed.)

My wife and I were shocked. So much said in so few words. We "meditated," caught our breath.

And so much unsaid! Here was a person who believed in her feelings, who followed her feelings — who *lived* her feelings. And what a tragedy . . .

Her feelings were gods that needed only to beckon to be followed. "If you have courage, follow me," they said. And she followed because she is a woman of courage.

I then began to see her as a victim of the so-called Human Potential Movement, or Growth Movement, which caught up thousands of middle class people (including myself) in a wave of enthusiasm that was so desperately needed to counter the doldrums of the Vietnam War and the blahs of consumerism.

The Growth Movement was far more than that of course. It was more than a "counter": it made — and still makes — an important contribution to our culture, to the very way in which so many of us now live our lives. The new focus of psychology on growth rather than disease; the awakening interest in *feeling* and *being* (as opposed to possessing); the new understanding of the human being as a body-mind amalgam; the new awakening to the intuitive and spiritual capabilities of all people are "just" some of its contributions.

But there have been deficits too — blind alleys, fads, distortions. A major distortion has been the *primacy* placed on feelings. A complete reversal occurred for many: from "uptight" to "hang loose." Now people could say anything and do anything as long as "real" feelings impelled them. The main question was: What are you *really* feeling?

And (in the thousands of encounter groups that proliferated) once you knew what you were feeling you "stayed with it" and "went with it." Those were the catchwords . . .

What a disaster for so many! The marriages, the families, the relationships broken because someone had a "righteous" feeling...The psyches scarred because someone projected his/her own anger on another in an encounter group or outside one...And the hurts still pile up because of a fundamental misunderstanding.

I think of the marriages I know — now smashed because one of the partners had been "liberated" by a therapy and so found the courage to surface long-smoldering resentments which, they felt, could not be healed through patient and loving listening. As if a disturbing behavior pattern (it takes two to create one!)would vanish in a subsequent relationship. For, of course, we take ourselves along in whatever relationship we form . . .

I also think of the encounter groups I have participated in that so traumatized me before I realized that I was not responsible for other people's malice and anger. On several occasions I required extensive discharge to heal the hurts from a "therapy" group.

For the patent, palpable truth is that FEELINGS ARE MEANT TO BE FELT, NOT NECESSARILY FOLLOWED! Feelings are not good per se; nor are they bad per so. They are simply meant to be felt. Only our intelligence can determine whether a feeling need be felt *and* followed.

Only intelligence can determine whether a followed feeling would foil or facilitate our rational goals and purposes. Only our intelligence can determine whether our feelings are servants or saboteurs. It is the function of intelligence to decide whether a feeling is congruent with our purposes or discordant.

Feelings are *not* gods. The dictum — you are your feelings — is a fallacy. We have many feelings that are not at all worthy of us. But we must take responsibiity for them, we must "own" them. Who would deny, for example, that feelings of despair and self-denigration (that might even approach suicidal dimensions) need to be discharged rather than followed? Who would deny that the "anger" we perpetrate on ourselves and others is almost invariably an unconscious disguise for fears, griefs, and blind spots we cannot face in ourselves? How often are our jealousies in an intimate relationship the projections of our own unvoiced and unmet needs in that relationship?

Furthermore we rarely grapple with *one* feeling. Feelings are parts of a continuum, a flow from one to the other. Which one do we choose to "go with"?

The key to that answer resides in our intelligence: in our commitment to the kind of Self, to the kind of human being we deep-down know we really are . . . underneath the strata of hurts that have been laid on us in our lives.

Yes, it's a matter of faith and trust, and our hypothesis of the intelligent, loving, cooperative, creative, joyous human being often *feels* fatuous and simplistic. But remember: cynicism derives from feelings too!

Never have we seen this fail: When human beings insist on full humanity, the negative feelings blocking that realization will discharge away to reveal the resplendant self.

It is difficult for *all of us* to acknowledge, since our culture is so damaging, that the natural human state is zestful. Not that we are positing a rosy-hued life without struggle and heartache; on the contrary we shall always have that, but we can struggle with buoyant affirmation once we feel our essential being, once we have sloughed off enough distressful feelings to sense our inner core . . .

Discharge will occur before, after, or even during a positive rational action that is challenging an habitual negative feeling. The point is that rational behavior is in no way a contradiction to an awareness of feelings. In fact, it stimulates such awareness. We can move rationally in the world *even though aware of negative feelings pulling at us to do the opposite* – and then release those feelings *when we are able to do so.* All of us have done — and continue to do — that as a matter of course!

For example, if we find ourselves in an awfully tight spot on the freeway, we generally don't panic first — we make the right maneuver and then perhaps pull over on the shoulder to shake and sweat and laugh the fear away until we feel centered again.

Or if we feel inadequate to do a job we know we must do, we "supervise" the feeling as best we can but do the job — and get on with the business of living. In practice all of us have learned to distinguish our selves from our feelings. Even those who worship at their altar must do that most of the time in order to survive!

How do we know whether a feeling is rational or not? Generally, of course, you do. Generally you can instantaneously correlate the results of following a feeling with its effect on your personal goals and with its appropriateness to the qualities of the undistressed human: intelligent, creative, loving, zestful.

But if we don't know, we counsel on it: with a friend or professional counselor (or with your friend-in-residence identified in our chapter on self-counseling). We talk it out, we feel it out, we act it out with someone other than the person who could be victimized by an inappropriate *restimulated* feeling sprung up from the past.

Why *restimulated*? Because suppressed feelings are like dynamic electric charges that can immediately connect (and explode!) — often when people and/or conditions are just barely similar to those existent when the original hurt occurred. For example, I am the perfect father type: in my 60's, with totally grey hair, and with occasionally an irrepressible penchant for "wisdom." And how often in therapy groups I have led has that grey hair been the lightning rod that attracted rage crackling out of the past from people had barely met minutes before — because I reminded them of their father.

In short, feelings don't think; nor are they supposed to. But we can. Moreover they are a challenge and an opportunity to shed light on a past that for some reason prevented them from surfacing appropriately. If you have the counseling opportunity, use it!

Anger — or what purports to be anger — is the most dangerous restimulated feeling because it can hurt, maim, or kill — emotionally or literally. It is also the most misunderstood emotion, for it wears many guises and carries the freight of other less comfortable feelings — namely fear and grief.

Thus it took me thirty years after my father's death to realize that my enduring "anger" at him was caused by my feeling that he had never blessed me — so that once I experienced the damnable hurt of feeling unblessed, my love for him came through and we have been close ever since. Thirty years of anger can be quite crippling . . .

Actually there are two angers. The common one is really closer to what we mean by frustration. If we are continually prevented from satisfying a need, we become frustrated ("angry") and if that frustration develops a sufficiently intense pressure we have rage (great "anger"). It can be taken as an axiom that rage is always a restimulated feeling, although its immediate provocation may indeed be angering or frustrating. If triggered therefore, its object will be a victim, a scapegoat, rather than someone who has received a useful communication. Rage needs to be discharged — not triggered — no matter how righteous it feels, since it is bound to be an overreaction.

Rage creates the "motiveless" crimes we read about in the newspapers — the "senseless" killings of innocent people. It destroys children battered by parents "beside themselves" with oceanic feelings. All it takes is a trigger . . .

Rage is piled-up frustration and/or anger that could have been useful at its inception; but its suppression and festering have caused it to be dangerous. Here is the key — the secret — to useful anger. At its inception it is a beautiful feeling indeed. It is not hurtful and it is miraculous in its efficacy. "True" anger is righteous without any disastrous side-effects. It lights up like a match — suddenly; flares intensely to reveal an important aspect of a personality; then dies almost immediately, with no negative reaction either in the "sender" or the "receiver". On the contrary, "true" anger creates a shared human opening between people...

Righteous anger is a way of saying "Stop! I've had enough!" It could be enough coddling, enough avoidance, enough criticism. Or it could be a social or political manifestation: enough oppression, enough violence (as we saw in the spontaneous demontrations caused by the killing of Martin Luther King Jr.)

Since anger is one of the few respected feelings in our culture — especially among men — it will often "encapsulate" the less respectable emotions of fear and grief but continue to wear the guise of anger until it discharges in shaking and tears. For example, we might be hurt if someone we care about does not invite us to a party we dearly want to attend — but we will be "furious" at the slight. And — especially among fighting boys — how marvelously does "anger" cinch up the fear of defeat and hurt while wearing the face of an avenging hero. Fear, indeed, is the least welcomed intruder in the manly breast.

We hope you have not sensed our implicit argument to be that feelings themselves are suspect, for in truth they are the all-encompassing medium that colors and flavors our life. To deny them would be to deny life. But to give them a will and destiny of their own would also deny life. We encourage positive feelings and the discharge of negative ones — but never the suppression of any feelings. Once again: FEELINGS ARE MEANT TO BE FELT, NOT NECESSARILY FOLLOWED.

The commitment we are talking about requires that we learn to *disidentify* from all feelings — surely the negatives — until we decide they are enhancing. For example, when you say, "I *am* tired," you really mean, "I *feel* tired." (Something exciting could occur and your tiredness would be gone!)

Or when you say, "I *am* angry," you really mean, "I *feel* angry." (*Am* and *feel* are worlds apart. With *am* you're stuck; with *feel* you have a variety of options.)

Nor, incidentally, are you your desires or your intellectual notions — worthy though they might be.

We are *awarenesses* that transcend all identifications. Our unique selves interconnect and interanimate with all other selves and with the universe. Our "boundaries" are limitless.

We can direct feelings like symphony conductors in order to connect, unite, expand, and grow with the oneness rather than allow ourselve to be slaves to our past.

In that way and with time joy will preside over our lives — even in struggle. *That* feeling — of joy in struggle — all of us can willingly follow!

THE WORLD OF THE BODY

Health becomes creative force as we embody the earth.

Exhaustion

Not long ago I ran into two men who live on the edge. Call them what you will, they'll be apt to acknowledge your label — outcasts, derelicts, bums, winos. What drew me to them is that I recognized one of them from third grade. We had played together, ran together for a whole year. The bond was still there.

And it was an opportunity to go way back and remember those childhood days with fondness. But then they recalled someone who had died, that I hadn't known. Somehow, hesistantly, I asked what he had died of, and they both looked at me with surprise as my friend finally explained (as if to a child), "Exhaustion, man, exhaustion."

I have since thought about that diagnosis often. I know you won't find it in hospital charts or autopsy reports or even in conversations of most "straight" people — but isn't that what we all die of, exhaustion? All the medical and psychological terminology of mortality simply describes aspects and conditions of exhaustion.

We die daily of exhaustion. Every day we function with the same program, the same compulsions, the same habits, we die an inch to exhaustion. Every day we exist in our special haze, our familiar film, our unique bubble, we die an inch to exhaustion. When we go to sleep so tired we cannot sleep but only lie there, we lie in exhaustion. And when we awaken to the same myriad concerns that trouble our sleep, we face the day in exhaustion.

Our way of life feeds exhaustion: the competition not with the self but with others; the stress on output over inner need; so that as a consequence we deplete our resources to exhaustion.

It's true that all of us have the inner urge toward organismic balance; yet the lack of cultural traditions that acknowledge the deeper places in our heart, and even our customary ways of relieving exhaustion, confound the problem so that we can no longer recognize its very presence. We are so used to running on mental energy, emotional excitement, and stimulating thoughts and foods that even when not in the workaday world we whip our bodies to continue the show; even our precious moments after work and on weekends and vacation are subject to the same stresses Searching for the unexhausting place exhausts us the more.

Surely if we had a gigantic invisible movie camera filming an average day in our lives — peering through walls, floors, ceilings into alleys and freeways; offices, factories, and supermarkets; bedrooms, bathrooms, and bars — for a full twenty-four hours, it would become manifest that we are a country that runs on drugs in our mad search for relaxation.

They are the modern way to deny exhaustion: when we are too tired to sleep, we take a pill; too tired to move, another; too tense to cope, still another. And if it's not pills, it's coffee, cigarettes, alcohol, cocaine, heroin, or another drug of preference. Like a ferris wheel we go round and round until we spend our tickets — and then we turn sick.

It's as if the body with its special wisdom knows that there is one chance for legitimate rest and so plays its trump card — sickness. Now at last we can accept "doing nothing" — as if resting, thinking, and dreaming were nothing! But there is another lure in sickness too: we can be cared for by others and we can even ask for attention without embarrassment. It even promises special bonus for some, for it can be a time for a new inner audit, an assessment of the personal economy, and a new re-evaluation with different priorities and emphases emerging.

But options narrow as our bodies grow older in the long cyclic struggle of stimulation and enervation so that sickness eventually becomes more serious, and exhaustion goes deeper. Formerly the expression of deep tiredness, now it records the malfunction of vital organs and glands.

It is at this point that true regeneration, true healing, a real reorganization of energy patterns, needs to be facilitated for a return to health; but there are virtually no provisions for such a reorientation. There is neither the time nor the place nor the cultural "ceremony" for such regeneration (After all, medication has removed the symptoms and the patient is now well).

In any case, economic compulsions bar the door to retreat, reassessment, and genuine recovery. Despite the new growth movement and a greater awareness of the limitations of a spend-and-enjoy philosophy, economic pressures on most people remain a constant factor perpetuating life-styles that create sickness. Yet it's not that simple, for even those who could get in touch with their creative power are stopped by the stimulation-enervation patterns they have integrated into their coping mechanisms.

Moreover, the incredible paradox is that all the therapies in the healing arts — biological as well as psychological — generally do not respond to the human aspirations that could finally shatter patterns leading to — a dead end. For, in order for true healing to occur, a new union with our life force, with our creative powers — with God, Great Spirit, call it what you will — must be experienced in order to short-circuit the dead end. And here most therapies are silent.

Yet we must reunite with our essence, with our loving selves, with our selves needing love, with our spark of creativity, or else all the regimens and all the techniques and all the therapies ultimately become dead ends too. The only lasting way to dissipate the exhaustion inherent in our way of life is the daily meeting with the creative force in our being which can reanimate our natural cycles of tension and relaxation — thought and feeling, work and play, effort and rest. (Even these cycles can become mechanical exercises unless love and joy suffuse them so that they seem to merge.)

Unfortunately, there is no instant remedy for exhaustion. Discharge of feelings will help enormously. (See Chapter 2)   Holistic nutritional practices will also help enormously. (See Chapter 6 .) But even the best of practices can also become chores, pressures, rites, meaningless idols — and so, exhausting. Exhaustion is subtle. It sneaks up on one slowly, imperceptibly. Only the daily attunement with our center can ward off the shadow.

Subtle also is the goal, for it is not placidity; the cure is not a tradeoff of excitement for sameness. On the contrary, when we are not exhausted we have more energy to give to life. Balance is the key, and a balanced awareness can only be actualized when we are attuned to the cycles of nature, to the bio-rhythms of our organism. There is a time for rapid movement, and for easy motion; for sleeping five hours a night, or twelve; for sowing seeds, or gathering in; for solitude, or outgoing. The key is our subtle sense of timing, so that we don't eat the same diet all year round, or stay indoors when blossoms are filling the air with their fragrance.

Perhpas the key is that there is no key but an in-touchness with reality; and reality is ever -changing — so how could there be an ANSWER.

But there *is* an infinity of beginnings — and we begin when we become aware of our own exhaustion or help others with theirs, and by so doing learn to exhaust exhaustion. We begin when we are in touch; for exhaustion, if it means anything, means being out of touch.

The beginning is in the living of our Selves. When we do that, there are no endings.

The Ceremony Of Hope

Disease is an opportunity! It is a ceremony. It is discovery, purification, and renewal. It is a pilgrimage to our inner temple where our essence abides. It is an invitation to healing — if we would heed it. It is the most magnificent healing ceremony ever created. It is our opportunity to renew life. It is a ceremony of hope.

We are called to it by our master of ceremonies — our own spirit. It is a call to purify, to be renewed, to cleanse, to breathe deeply, to illumine the shadows of our hearts, to silence the maddening echoes of our minds, to break cultural shackles — to fell the walls of Jericho.

We are called to that ceremony named disease to be released from the incessant pressures and worries of our life and to become aware of the plaguing oppressor or victim roles we play. We are called to acknowledge the place of love deep in our being. We are called to that ceremony named disease before the altar of the heart in the temple of the body to experience our inner reality removed from its husk of daily life. We are called to the one ceremony — with birth and death — that all humans everywhere share in common.

But how bitter it is for most to be ill! It is almost an accusation of weakness, or perverseness. Don't we know that we can't be cared for properly? Don't we know the hardships we'll cause? The bills to be paid, the added work to be done, the worries to be borne?

In truth, few can even economically afford the space to learn from disease. Yet even for them the true causes of disease are rarely unveiled. If people could see what is depleting them — their denatured food, the poisoned air, the dehumanizing economic pressures, their alienating sexual and social roles — they would do something, and there would be a tremendous shakeup of our total way of life.

But the forces that control the media and teach our young, that process the food, that indoctrinate us into our way of life, are strong. And unfortunately our medical system, advanced as it may be in emergency life-support situations, is amazingly deficient in dealing with the healing needs of daily life. Rather than paticipating in the healing journey, more often than not treatment suppresses therapeutic symptoms or removes ailing parts. Little faith is shown in self-healing biological processes.

Moreover, because we have never been taught a faith in life itself, fear prevents us from realizing that the manifestations of disease are the organism's healing response; and so our minds indict the body and thus prevent the re-evaluation of a pathogenic lifestyle. Often a conversation much like the following takes place during illness:

MIND: I do not feel well.
BODY: I know — am trying to do something about it.
MIND: Oh yeah? *You* are the reason I am feeling bad.
BODY: You've got that backwards, my friend.
MIND: You don't know anything about directions. You're just a machine and you've broken down.
BODY: I am alive — I am no machine — what you call breakdown is service, an opportunity.
MIND: You think you know so much.
BODY: I don't think...(mind interrupts.)
MIND: I noticed that. You're primitive.
BODY: My sole work is to do everything in my power to insure your survival.
MIND: Then why in the hell do you get sick?
BODY: To protect you.
MIND: From what?
BODY: From yourself.
MIND: Shut up! I've had enough...

With all the brilliance of the mind, it often takes a superior and elititst position to the body, unaware that they are both compounded of the same physical stuff and that the body is endowed with billions of cells manifesting an intelligence and wisdom and intuition that are bulwarks for its survival.

Regardless of personal and cultural blindness, disease originates in the way we live. It is not some foreign invader set out to do us in. Furthermore, the expression of disease, its symptoms, its manifestation of imbalance, are no less than ways in which the innate intelligence of our organism its attempting to heal itself.

Disease is a result and not the cause of our disturbance. If we could observe, we would see that it comes when our energy flow is not honoring some primary level of our being. It comes when we lose hope. when our creativity is drained, when we have been shocked, when we experience loss. It comes when our body is saturated with poisons that our liver and glands are too exhausted to process.

It is a warning that we are not fulfilling our needs. Its message is actually one our innate intelligence creates to save ourselves from destruction, and its expressions are simply the ways our organism provides to cleanse, to rebuild and renew, and to rest. Our organismic intelligence, always at play in the dance of life and death, expresses itself most dramatically when it attempts to awaken us to our true needs through the language of disease.

And its most gripping current statement is cancer, for cancer is not only a disease of the person but of the social and economic fabric, and therefore its appropriate healing response must be total. Frightening though it is, we must regard cancer as our great teacher come to awaken us from chronic disregard of our natural beings. We must embrace its dire message, for it too is a ceremony of hope!

But it will require an entire shift of consciousness and lifestyle to cure, for cancer in our bodies is a reflection of cancer in the water, air, and earth; of cancer of the spirit, reflecting its despairs, its mute losses, its alienation from the body. But its presence can awaken us to abandon our present cultural posture in order to honor our innate intelligence and the essential oneness.

But, unfortunately, the greatest successes of the medical profession have been gained in dealing with microbial epidemics through identification of the "enemy" germ and subsequent use of mass hygienic practices to eliminate it — so that they still insist on viewing cancer as an enemy that has infiltrated the battle lines and seized control of our cells and tissues and therefore must be ir- radiated, excised, and poisoned. even though the enemy is not a germ and will soon very likely "invade" the organism on a new frontier. With all their magnificent equipment, it slips through the lines undetected, because it comes from within!

The reason is that it is a disease of being, of our existence, of the way we exchange our energy for economic goods, of the way we relate to ourselves and others, of the way we love — and hate. *Cancer is the result of the chronic suppression of previous "ceremonies" intended to cleanse, heal, and renew:* unacknowledged ceremonies that could only be "affirmed" through cancer. Cancer is the final ceremonial escalation.

Since we live in a culture of fragmented consciousness, since we are separated from the products we make and from those who help us make them, since we are separated from ourselves through consumerism, drugs, and competition, since we are even sepa- rated from those we love through anxiety and fear — it is a won- der that cancer has not struck in even greater proportions, though it already visits one out of four Americans!

Thus cancer provides us with the supreme example of a disease that calls for a healing ceremony that will transform our entire way of life and for a response therefore that will engage our responsibi- lity not only for ourselves but for everyone on the planet, since this is a planetary ceremony — but more fundamentally, since our being is of the earth and therefore is one with all other human beings. It is my profound hope and prayer that its dire call will be a catalyst to alter our present martial attitudes toward disease — so that perhaps sometime in the not too distant future we will view cancer as the crisis that saved our lives.

Then we will see all disease as a ceremony of hope, as a rite of unification for our spirits so that the blossom of human creation can flourish.

Nutrition:

HONORING THE SPIRIT IN MATTER

An Overview

Breath and life, food and peace, seed and psyche are all connected in the great chain of life. And so it is that to understand the way food works — when we must eat and when we need fast, what we must eat and when we need stop — is a relatively simple matter, yet reflects deep philosophical concerns. Our physical body is worthy of this concern, for it contains an amazing spiritual laboratory wherein the nutrients of the earth are exalted. The earth and the body interpenetrate. I, for one, take my body to my earthly Mother for care and healing. I shun man-made panaceas that disregard our source of life.

After nearly a decade-and-a-half of intense research and experimentation, I want to share a nutritional viewpoint that honors the biological, sociological, psychological, and spiritual realms; a viewpoint that credits the findings of biochemical sciences but still understands the importance of living foods; that participates in the values of rational scientific efforts but also in the experiential wisdom of native peoples all over the globe. It is a viewpoint that believes optimal food comes from healthy soil and that inorganic chemicals cannot compensate for its deficiencies. Most important, it is a nutritional viewpoint that facilitates the conscious transformation of matter to spirit, of conditioning to freedom and of despair to faith.

Only the heart can truly understand nutrition, for though, like a river, this science flows through the fields of biochemistry, physiology, genetics, psychology, agriculture, and sociology, its destination is the ocean of life; and the life spirit cannot be investigated in the laboratory. For we are not mechanisms, we are organisms; we are not simply burners of fuel, we are vitalizers of fuel; we are not flesh run by brain but flesh that is brain — brain that is attuned to the cellular reality of our being.

Optimal nutrition can only be obtained when the pulse of life is assimilated into that being by meeting the biological requirements of our cells. What is known as metabolism is the meeting of the pulse of life with our cells; that is why we can understand nutrition at its most basic level if we can envision our cells being responsive to the life current that reciprocally interpenetrates the earth and every cell of the living organism.

Nutritionists therefore must be open to "receive" the vitality of the earth through attunement with its elements. But they cannot stop there. Their main function is to perceive the progress of those elements through the chain of life, not only as biochemical substances but as products of human celebrations: the harvest, the hunt, the catch, the gather.

It is now time for the nutritionist to step outside the laboratory into real life to meet the farmers in their laboratory so that together they can fulfill their mutual responsibility for optimal nutrition. It is time the nutritionist acts on the realization that the way a plant or animal is raised determines its vitality. It is time the nutritionist becomes aware that human creative powers can now properly feed all of humanity — but that political forces primarily are preventing this historic consummation. It is time, in other words, that the nutritional sciences become the vehicle for a holistic consciousness that could feed a now fractured world.

The Way of Nurturance

It is such a consciousness that develops what I call the way of nurturance — a way that would guarantee all humans their birthright activities of peaceful construction, food production, childrearing, healing, and artistic creation, and that would particularly focus on insuring a reservoir of vital nutrients for all peoples.

It is a way that would guarantee not only an adequate supply of nucleic acids, minerals, proteins, vitamins, trace elements, carbohydrates, and friendly bacteria but would also aim at simplifying production and distribution so that we could begin to rely (once again!) on locally produced food that need no longer be "preserved," frozen, stabilized, fortified, enchanced, colored, or gassed.

Tragically, our agriculture, our food industry, and our medical establishments are obsessed with a chemical consciousness rather than a nutritional awareness. Chemicals can never biologically nourish nor insure our physical integrity; though, of course, there are situations and conditions that warrant their careful use, in fact when it would be criminal not to use them.

But to use them unawarely is to deepen the current health crisis. Even when useful in emergencies — as nutrients, as biologically absorbed substances, they always leave imbalance, be it in the soil or in the blood. Their omnipresence can only denote the fragmentation of our awareness through economic pressure and its consequence, the separation of the laboratory from daily life. They are notorious in so-called junk foods, but they are more insidious in basic foods — such as vegetables and fruit, livestock and grain — because these are the foundation of our national diet, and yet we know that they impede the vital digestive exchange from food cell to human cell.

In California alone over 400 million pounds of insecticide are used annually! Whether we are hermits or food junkies, those chemicals reside in our bones; therefore they also disturb our spiritual body, for we are all one. That is why involvement with food requires ultimately a total awareness that will impel even non-political people to take a stand against agribusiness. We will inevitably move toward life and support practices that nurture life!

That is why a change in outlook for large numbers of people is my most cherished hope, for a new nutritional consciousness can accomplish far more than even the individual "miracles" of naturopathic healers. It is vastly encouraging to know that that outlook must also be a social and political expression of the way of nurtrance. The path toward new priorities starts with the awakening of the human spirit for a new co-relationship with the food that gives it flesh. It is an awakening toward oneness.

The result and the promise of this change of outlook, this new nutritional consciousness, this way of nurturance, is the experience of being grounded, of feeling our roots, of feeling the earth and our dependency upon it, of feeling therefore our universality and our fellowship with all people who are rooted on this planet Earth.

There is an inherent urge in the human being to ground, to feel and resonate with biological reality, and thus — to bloom. But if that urge is thwarted, we tend to suppress the resultant anxiety by "somaticizing" it with strong physical sensations from drugs or alcohol, loveless sex, and overeating or overinvolvement in the digestive process.

Therefore, the rational human goal is to be so awarely grounded that we respond *consciously* to the sensations of hunger and love that power our primal pulse in order to fulfill the creative urge *in harmony with all other beings.*

Three Stages Of Growth

We will look at the path to good nutrition in three major stages. First will be awareness. Awareness that we may have poor nutrition and need to change it. The second is the transition stage. In the transition , we identify those foods that are harmful to us and also those that are helpful. With this knowledge, we can construct a much healthier diet than what we have been using. Most people will be satisfied with the improvement in their health that will come from having gone through this transition stage. There are many people, however, that want to put a great deal more effort into watching their daily diet. For them, we have added a third stage — the stabilization. But first we need to be aware:

Awareness

First Stage

There is so little that one can say about awareness, and yet it encompasses all the stages; for without it we cannot proceed. And even at the highest level it is possible to regress — unawarely! Awareness is the essential ingredient...

What is it then nutritionally? It is the ability to observe our own conditioning in the realm of diet — and that is no simple matter . For we have been trained with the sugar water imbibed at our very birth into a dietary mode that seems completely natural even though it is a relatively *recent* massive experiment to induce consumption of highly processed foods created by profit-making technology, advertised by amazingly powerful media, and endorsed by a prestigious medical establishment.

It is the ability to observe what happens when we stop using sugar, when we stop drinking coffee, when we stop using alcohol, when we stop consuming denatured bread, etc.

At this stage of the awakening we need not permanently stop, but we do need to test for a sufficient length of time the results of stopping so that we can begin the awareness process. We need to experience in our own bodies the discomforts of withdrawal from sugar, alcohol, coffee, and the hundreds of other chemicalized substances that comprise the popular diet. And then we need to resume consuming them so that we can advance in the process of awareness by noting what they do in our own "laboratory."

That is the way we become observers of our own conditioning. And that is the way therefore we discover we have choices. Awareness becomes the process that continually supplies us with the new choices we need to confront in order to make our diet *our own*.

It is the process that will enable us to understand personally — literally. — the significance of a recent report of a U.S. Senate subcommittee on nutrition concluding that one-third of the degenerative diseases in our society would be eliminated if the American diet included more complex carbohydrates, vegetables, fruit, and non-animal protein instead of its vast emphasis on white sugar, animal fats, and refined carbohydrates.

The report was immediately attacked by the food industry so that its influence will not be great. But what is encouraging is that the large body of testimony validates what naturopathic doctors, chiropractors, and nutritionists have been saying for seventy-five years.

If we actually know what happens in our own bodies when we use processed food, then our awareness potential will also be capable of supporting us to eat well *consistently*; and that is vital, for consistency is the prime requisite for nutritional grounding. It is essential to understand that no crash diet, exercise program, fast, or vitamin regimen can create biochemical health. Health is "done" slowly, laboriously, undramatically. That is why awareness is necessary to confront our conditioning so that we will eat consistently well day in and day out — neither too sweet nor too sour, neither too much protein nor too little, etc. Then consistency itself will help create a new awareness: that "quiet," simple natural foods give a pleasure of their own, a pleasure marred by neither "highs" nor lows nor withdrawal symptoms.

Transition

Second Stage

After the awareness stage comes the transition. After experiencing the roller coaster of our chemically "fortified" diet, there comes a new level of eating and being on which we can profit by and gain pleasure from our previous discoveries. Now we will naturally eliminate foods harmful to our organism and include those that are nourishing. Eventually we will begin to embrace the simple basic foods.

Yet during the transition there is no revolution in diet. We still eat — more or less — what we've eaten, but now they are *whole* foods, and if at all possible, organically raised and thoughtfully prepared. If we want to eat french toast for breakfast, we use whole grain bread and naturally produced eggs.

The transition is not the time for giving up foods unless you have discovered they give you up. It is a time for becoming attuned to whole foods in the various food groups. It is a time for living unaddicted to the hypertensive American diet. It is a time that provides needed space before moving into the stabilization stage — if we so choose. It is a time for liberation from our conditioning.

Perhaps these guidelines will help you in your transition:

1. While improving the quality of your food, still honor your dietary upbringing and cultural traditions.
2. Harmonize your diet with your lifestyle. If you live in a stressful urban environment, your nutritional needs will be greater — so eat accordingly.
3. Although the transition diet encompasses a variety of foods, it is still beneficial to establish order in the eating patterns. The body functions best with order.
4. The craving for sweets is caused by lifestyle and/or emotional constrictions. In terms of diet — pay attention to the B vitamins.
5. Continuous craving and hunger often indicates a deficiency of nucleic-acid-rich food. Replenish! (See Proteins, pp 69-73.)
6. Depending on your beliefs, pray and/or commune in your fashion with the oneness before eating. Then chew well.

Foods to Avoid in the Transition

To reinforce your awareness, the following list of cautionary foods is included as a useful reference:

1. *White sugar*

White sugar is a non-food whose main effect is the rapid elevation of the blood-sugar level. It does this because it requires virtually no digestion and so immediately enters the bloodstream, producing a stimulation invariably followed by depression. This roller-coaster effect is very wearing on the organism.

Another side effect of sugar consumption is a gradual deterioration of the pancreas and the consequent depletion of its vital enzymes, inducing a host of complications including diabetes, hypoglycemia, and cancer, as well as psychological confusion caused by glucose starvation of the nerves and brain.

Consumption of white sugar inevitably supplants nutritious foods that are needed by our organism. Furthermore, white sugar is produced with large amounts of pesticides and harmful chemicals that give it its "pure white" look.

2. *Refined grains and foods containing them*

Refined grain is a food robbed of its vital substance much as a human body robbed of its heart. The essential vitamins and minerals are discarded with only the starch left. Refined grain acts like a glue in the stomach, thus blocking entry of important nutrients. Regular consumption of refined grain cause liver damage and a whole range of metabolic disturbances.

3. *Salt*

Except for small amounts of (sea) salt during pregnancy, the body is provided with ample sodium and other minerals from vegetables, herbs, water, sea weed and kelp. Salt is a stimulant. It elevates blood pressure and "whips" the adrenal glands to secrete. It interferes with the elimination of metabolic waste products, irritating the delicate tubules in the kidneys, the prostrate gland in the male, and the womb in the female.

According to Dr. Henry Bieler[1], it can, under certain conditions, also irritate the brain through the diffusable electrolytes entering the cerebrospinal fluid. Moreover, Dr. Max Gerson[2], one of the pioneers of non-toxic cancer therapy, believes the overconsumption of salt to be a contributing cause of cancer.

[1] See "Food Is Your Best Medicine", Henry Bieler M.D. Vintage Books, 1965
[2] See "A Cancer Therapy - Results of Fifty Cases" , Max Gerson M.D., Duro Books, 1958

4. *Processed dairy products*

In the great design of nature, milk is intended to pass from nipple to mouth. The farther from this ideal the more harmful it is to the organism. Heating, drying, freezing, and otherwise altering raw milk make it problematic except in survival circumstances (famine, disaster, mountaineering).

One out of six human beings does not produce adequate enzymes to digest milk properly. For the other five who do, however, *locally produced* milk still remains a reliable source of easily digestible protein.

You will be especially fortunate if you can obtain goat's milk, for it is far more digestible than cow's milk. Incidentally, goats convert feed into milk six times more efficiently than cows.

5. *Chemically fed livestock*

Many nations around the globe will not buy U.S. produced meat because of its high levels of hormones, chemicals, and fat. If you do eat meat, it is important to purchase only naturally raised animals and learn how to use this food properly. (See page 86 in Stabilization section.)

6. *Artifically produced eggs*

Chickens that are kept awake with stimulants twenty-two hours daily and prevented from scratching the ground for greens and insects cannot produce healthy eggs. Naturally raised eggs are used in the transition stage. They can be eaten either soft-boiled or poached. If raw, use only the yolk (it's fine in a blended drink).

7. *Coffee*

Coffee is another non-food produced at the expense of traditional agriculture in third world countries. People who grow coffee commonly exist in a state of permanent malnutrition. They should be growing food crops for their own consumption.

Coffee is a stimulant that whips the adrenal glands to secrete. After years of use it will damage the liver and kidneys. (It takes about seven years for its acids to clog the kidneys — a lifeline organ.)

Not so incidentally, many of the most lethal pesticides that have even been banned in the U.S. are *exported* to coffee-producing countries which return them in our national beverage!

8.   *Soft drinks*

Soft drinks not only fill the system with harmful chemicals, sweetners, flavor-enhancers, caffeine, etc., but also leach vital minerals from the body.

9.   *Alcohol*

Commercially produced alcohol is loaded with chemicals also. So not only are we depleted by its emotional effects but also by its nitrates, insecticides, and bacterial growth inhibitants. Those with a particular psychological affinity for alcohol should aim to stop its use entirely. (We know that's not easy. Therefore, we recommend counseling on the distress that comes up as you cut down.)

10.   *Seasonings*

The problem with *most* seasonings is that they mask the taste and stimulate the taste buds so that we eat more than we need. Properly prepared natural food needs very little adornment. Many seasonings — such as black pepper — actually irritate the delicate linings of the stomach.

11.   *Refined oils*

Refined and processed oils are a major contributor to cardio-vascular disease. Since they are generally heated in food preparation, they become even more detrimental. Hydrogenated oils — closer to plastic than food — actually coat the system with a toxic residue.

High quality vegetable oils — such as olive, sesame, corn, safflower, and sunflower — are rich in such necessary nutrients as linoleic acid and vitamin F and in important elements like calcium and phosphorus.

Coming Home

The way of nurturance that develops and expands during the transition eventually arrives at a mature phase which can be described as both an affirmation of the healing properties of basic foods and of humanity's common need for these foods. It's as if we have returned to our center, to our natural home.

But before we discuss the properties of these foundation foods, it is essential that we understand the reasons for having left home. When we do, it will become clear why it is so natural to return.

Why then did we? Basically because we did not have a strong enough national tradition (for a host of historical causes) to withstand — let alone guide — the burgeoning food industry as it took off with propulsive power to utilize a technology that saw vast benefit in using chemicals, standardization practices, and advertising techniques in order to command the national market. Perhaps if we had not been originally a nation of such diverse cultures, the protest would have been greater, though many did speak out. These were the grandmothers and grandfathers of our now strong ecological "movement".

Another key reason is related to the first. As our national economy was absorbed into mass corporate industry; as the railroad, then the automobile, then the airplane dominated our life; as the superhighway, the suburb, and the supermarket fixed their hold; and as movies, advertising, and television dominated our consciousness, we as a people were faced with great stress which we began to compensate for nutritionally. This was nirvana for the food trusts: they supplied the chemical boosts and buffers in their products while Americans gorged.

Yet food strikes back when used to satisfy non-biological needs. True, sweets are tempting because they are expansive, their taste lingers, and they are so soothing they seem a perfect specific for being stuck in an incessant drive for accomplishment or in holding patterns that deny emotional release. True, substances that whip our adrenals to get us "high", give us a lift, get us over the rough spots, (highly salted foods, overcooked proteins, chocolate, coffee, cola drinks, and even cortisone and antibiotics come to mind) are tempting if we are heavy with exhaustion. But food retaliates and has struck with a whole range of disorders and degenerative diseases that now "perplex" the medical establishment.

So once we become conscious of our conditioning during the nutritional awareness stage, it becomes clear why it is only natural that we return to the basics in the stage of transition — and we inevitably will if we seriously follow the way of nuturance. We do return home.

One brief caution before we credit our basic foods . . . It is important to realize that we cannot find "salvation" through dietary change. Salvation — if there be such — can only come from following the *various* ways of oneness and even then cannot be counted on. As a matter of fact, eating well might very likely intensify one's vulnerability and sensitivity by uncovering distressful feelings formerly suppressed by the ill-advised food. (It would be advisable in that case to "discharge" them. See chapter 2, for guidance.)

It is important to participate in the nutritional realm with a perspective that will free you from false hope while allowing you to experience the positive effects of dietary attunement.

Basic Foods for Transition

The basic nourishing foods we seek for our diet can be broken into four main catagories:

A) Protein
B) Whole Grains
C) Vegetables
D) Fruit

Let's look at each of these catagories starting with the most important — Proteins.

A — Proteins

Power creators of the healthy diet.

Proteins are made up of approximately twenty-two building blocks, called amino acids. Eight of these are considered essential. Foods that contain the essential amino acids are known as complete proteins; however, through the proper combining of foods at a meal, one can create complete protein.

Since protein is absolutely essential to the human organism, one should be wary of dietary experiments that advocate minimal protein intake. However, most Americans eat too much — often improperly prepared.

Such misuse contributes to a wide range of metabolic disorders. Excess protein stored in the tissues of the body results in what is known as overacidity and upsets nitrogen metabolism and our acid-base balance.

Protein foods are the most taxing on the digestive organs, and the residual compounds that result from their indigestion deplete glands and organs such as the liver, kidneys, and thyroid. The lack of energy so many people experience is often associated with over-consumption of the wrong kinds of protein.

It is also essential for the understanding of protein foods to realize that only *some* contain the nucleic acids that are crucial to health; and we must also be aware that the human body is composed of single cells, each alive through its own metabolism, each capable of regenerative processes that keep us alive.

Furthermore, the way our cells regenerate determines our health; however, regeneration can only be optimal if all necessary nutrients are present. If they are not, DNA and RNA — the nucleic acids — will be unable to complete their mission of transmitting vitality to the newly birthed cell.

The nucleic acids are found in some foods and can be synthesized by others. Therefore, these primary and auxiliary sources will be mentioned below.

Proteins for Our Transition

Here are seven excellent ways to get proteins.

(1)   A complete protein meal.

A combination of whole grains — such as millet, buckwheat, or sprouted wheat — with seeds, nuts, sprouts, or legumes and vegetables, (beets, onions, mushrooms, spinach) provides a complete nucleic-acid-rich protein meal.

(2)   Seeds and Nuts.

We advise combining these foods and then using them in moderation. They may also be soaked in water and germinated to facilitate digestion and create the nutrients associated with growing foods.

Sesame seeds —

High in calcium — twice as much as its phosphorus, an excellent proportion — they also contain inositol, choline, niacin, and vitamin E.

Sunflower seeds —

These are also rich in vitamin E and the B vitamins and are capable (along with the herb comfrey) of synthesizing vitamin B12.

Pumpkin seeds —

Generally discarded! They are rich in zinc and especially beneficial for bladder and kidney healing.

Almonds —
They are rich in phosphorus, copper, nitrilosides.

Walnuts —
The walnut is rich in vitamin B1 and iron.

Other nuts —
You will notice I did not mention peanuts or the imported seeds and nuts. Peanuts and peanut butter are generally more difficult to digest than the other nuts. If you must use them, mix them with other seeds and nuts (ground). The imported nuts (cashews, brazil nuts, etc.) generally are more difficult to digest, are associated with the big power politics of food; furthermore, they must be fumigated before entering the country.

(3)   Eggs.

Eggs from healthy chickens allowed to scratch on the ground and fed greens are an excellent protein source and rich in nucleic acids. They should be lightly cooked (poached or soft boiled is best). The raw egg yolk is perhaps the greatest medicine for rebuilding depleted adrenal glands. The white is not to be eaten raw for it depletes B vitamins.

(4)   Dairy Products.
Raw Milk —

This excellent source (used as a food, not a beverage!) of easily digestible protein (unless you're allergic) poses some problems. First off, there are personal and ecological considerations that need be dealt with individually.
Then there's the question of a fresh local source. I did not use dairy products for many years. Then I moved to a neighborhood where a woman who loves her goats and feeds them alfalfa and comfrey shares their milk with her neighbors. I began using it and have

found it a beneficial addition to my diet.

So if you have the source and the inclination, I recommend it. Although not brimming with nucleic acids, its whey does help in their synthesis. It will help you get what you need.

Yogurt —

Here is a food especially beneficial for its friendly bacteria that result from the culturing process. They are important when so many drugs, chemicals, and additives in the air and food destroy our intestinal flora. It also contains vitamin B12.

Cheese —

This dairy product is not an ideal food because of its fat, salt, and age. However, if one is active and well, small amounts can be used. In nutritional therapy it is definitely avoided.

(5) Beans.

Tofu (soybean curd) is an excellent way to eat beans. It is a lightly cooked product and some is now made from organically grown beans.

If you are active and healthy, other beans are a plausible option; however, if you have any digestive disturbance or general health problem, switch to more easily assimilated proteins.

(6) Meat.

As a nutritional psychologist it is my responsibility to work — if at all possible — with my clients' cultural attitudes toward food while attempting to improve their daily nutritional process. Yet it is my personal judgment that unless meat is organically produced it should not be used.

At the least — those who must have meat need to use it properly. Generally this means consuming it in smaller amounts and combining it with vegetables. (Please see How to Eat, pp. 85-86.)

(7)   Fish.

A fine nucleic-acid-rich protein. When lightly cooked, it is an easily digestible animal food.

B — Whole Grains

Power Sustainers of the Healthy Diet .

Whole grains maintain the proper blood-sugar balance by absorbing gradually into the blood stream, thus protecting the vital force of the organism. If we do not eat enough of these complex carbohydrates, we must use our protein as fuel — wasting organismic energy as well as the protein resources of the planet.

Here follow capsule descriptions of the important grains:

Brown Rice — Rich in minerals (sodium, potassium, phosphorus)

Millet —   An alkaline grain. — and a very digestible protein. Rich in nitrilosides.

Oats —   Rich in calcium and silicon.

Wheat —   Especially recommended in its sprouted state in which its gluten, difficult for many to digest, has been transformed into an easily digestible sugar.

Corn —   Rich in lecithin and provitamin A, and E. A good warm-weather grain.

Buckwheat — Rich in rutin, a component of vitamin C.

Barley —   Very soothing to the inner linings of the intestines. Rich in B vitamins.

C — Vegetables and Herbs:

Rejuvenating catalysts in the Basic Healthy Diet

Every food has its own powers, and the best way to learn them is to listen to their language in our body. The communication of plant cells with ours in the digestive process is especially subtle and demands close attention; but the "listening" will be rewarding because it promotes specific healing reactions. American Indians were acutely aware of this language, as were many nutritionists of the last century. Their discoveries have stood the test of time. It is also essential to bear in mind that greens are our source of chlorophyll, perhaps the most important substance in human nutrition.

Following are brief descriptions of the qualities of various plant groups. (Listings of some basic herbs can be found near the end of the stabilization section, p 91.)

Celery —   A highly benefical nerve food and an important source of organic sodium. It is highly endowed with calcium and potassium also. The leaves of celery contain a substance akin to insulin.

Parsley —   Noteworthy for fighting infection. It also helps maintain proper functioning of the thyroid gland and abounds in vitiman A.

Spinach —   A natural mine for the vital amino and nucleic acids, as well as iron and folic acid.

String Beans - Notable for their potassium content, they are a specific for all neutralizing diets and those aimed at restoration of the pancreas and liver.

Lettuce —   A calming food and rich in folic acid.

Chard —   Rich in sodium and minerals.

Zucchini —   A specific for the liver with its rich supply of organic sodium.

Beets — Build up red corpuscles in the blood and are an excellent bulk food high in vitamin C and potassium.

Carrots — Their juice approximates the constituents of mothers' milk. They increase resistance to colds and infection because of their supply of vitamins A and C. They also contain generous amounts of B, D, and E.

Winter Squash — A fine source of easily digestible carbohydrates blessed with vitamin A and rich in iron and magnesium.

Potatoes — (white, red and yams) All excellent winter foods rich in digestible carbohydrates and minerals.

Onions, Garlic — Vastly useful for fighting infections. Garlic is an incredible herb used for arthritis, high blood pressure and cancer. Both are sulphur-rich.

D. Fruit

Fresh fruit are a wonderfully beneficial and cleansing food. They contain, if properly ripened, essential vitamins and minerals in their nectar. It is always best to eat fruit that grow near your home since they bear special qualities suitable to *your* situation.

For example, the pineapple, a refrigerant, lowers the body temperature and is therefore good for a fever or for a tropics-dweller, but in cold weather is hardly helpful. Fruit are best eaten in season between meals, alone, or with dairy products. It is not good to eat fruit before a meal because they dilute and alkalinize digestive enzymes and secretions, making absorption of grain or protein foods more difficult.

Although fruit can be incredibly delightful and satisfying — truly the most gracious of nature's foods — they must be eaten carefully. For example, it is dangerous to make them a staple food (as some try to do) since their mild energy is insufficient to handle the heavy vibrations of our civilization. Moreover, they sensitize those who live on fruit in ways that are dangerous within our cultural context. So if you want to be a *frutarian*, find yourself a spot in paradise!

I have found the apple to be the safest and most versitile non-tropical fruit. Rich in such minerals as potassium and magnesium and high in vitamin C, it contains valuable digestive enzymes and can be eaten with vegetables. In fact, Dr. Max Gerson, the renowned cancer specialist used it extensively with carrot juice.

Fruit: Nature's Graces

Cherries —   Blood-purifying, rich in iron.

Figs —   Their regenerative powers are amazing (the seeds are the answer). Rich in iron, very alkaline.

Apricots —   One of the most amazingly delicious gifts of nature. Contains vitamin A.

Pears —   A specific for healing the gall bladder. Very soothing.

Limes, Lemons —   In small amounts early in the day they can be excellent toning foods.

Grapefruit —   An important cleansing food (See Recipes, "The Kind The People Eat," p. 96, for fruit-juice combination.)

Honey —   (We realize honey is not a fruit, but it seems to fit here.)Honey is used in the transition to replace sugar. In addition to being a wonderful food, it has antiseptic powers and is rich in trace minerals, manganese, and vitamin B12.

We have now surveyed the stage of transition, and so it would be useful to comment briefly on this part of the journey — to look back before we go on to the stabilization stage.

The major point is that if you are well and satisfied with your health you need not go on! — for you have already arrived at the traditional "good old balanced diet" that has fortified generations of healthy humans; it is my judgment, after years of working with all kinds of nutritional programs and therapeutic regimes, that if those in good health would just begin to live by foods in the transition they could maintain their health.

Stabilization

Third Stage

The stabilization is for those who want and need to go further. Perhaps the pressing reason is health: you may want to regain your vitality; or perhaps your digestion is poor; or else you might have chronic metabolic problems that could eventuate in serious dysfunction. Or perhaps you want to learn so that you can help others learn; and if that is so, you are probably also moved by the spirit of stabilization, which journeys beyond literal dietary matters to the broad ways in which we exchange energy with nature and with our fellow human beings on this planet. It is a movement toward oneness — to the spirit made flesh through foods harvested from nature by the labor and sacrifice of the farmer and the field worker.

If it is for health reasons you want to proceed, you will soon discover what foods really "work" for you since your consistency of eating will have given you the sensitivity not only to discover their general effects but also their specific features so that you will know when to eat them and how best to prepare them. Furthermore, you will learn how to correlate your diet with such factors as age, climate, occupation, exercise, sleep, sex, and stress. Finally, you will become receptive to the key factor of nutrition, oxygenation, which is the basis of all the vital processes and all rejuvenation programs.

In the stabilization we can creatively realize our relationships with food by following its connections to all facets of life: to the undernourished, to the Third World peasants who farm non-food export crops, to our almost lost food traditions, to the menace of chemicals and additives, but particularly to the inspiring bounty of nature! After all is said, we move on to the stabilization to be closer to Mother Nature, for she is our prime inspiration!

Perhaps these following guidelines for the diet of "working persons" at the stage of stabilization will furnish a useful preface to the ground we now need to survey. ("Working persons" in this context means those who pursue a particular calling and are active in the world *as it is*, while being aware of the spiritual and evolutionary aspects of their life.)

The Stabilization Diet for Working Persons

1. We become familiar with the three modes of the nutritional process: Purification, Rejuvenation, and Sustenance.

2. We are increasingly attuned to the energy potential of foods we eat and how our organism "meets" this energy.

3. We consider protein carefully. Our protein foods are either lightly cooked or raw.

4. We combine food thoughtfully.

5. Meals are simple and their timing is relevant to our real needs.

6. We learn to use such "power foods" as sprouts, nutritional yeast, vitamins, and fresh vegetable juices in our daily diet as well as in therapy.

7. We eat consistently well.

Three Modes of The Nutritional Process In Stabilization

Now we need to become familiar with the three modes of the nutritional process (Purification, Rejuvenation & Sustenance) so that we can learn to orchestrate them into our daily life.

Purification

Purification is an intense biological process that results from living for periods of time on a limited quantity — though a very high quality — of food, liquid, or water.

Since the body no longer need expend its energy on digesting and absorbing new increments of food habitually consumed at mealtimes, it concentrates its organismic force on the elimination of damaged and diseased cells and the re-establishment of new metabolic homeostasis.

Since this process is intense, it should take place in a peaceful environment, for it is not unlikely that the self will also confront simultaneously psychological poisons of self-disdain, greed, fear, hate, etc., that will surface when the foods we ordinarily use to suppress them are no longer present. The negative feelings need to be discharged as well. (See Chapter 2 for suggestions.) A musical ambiance is often appropriate for this ingathering of the body-mind. Inspirational books are also often helpful.

The safest substances to purify with are fresh vegetable juice, vegetable broths, herbal teas, or simple combinations of a few foods. (See Recipes for combinations beneficial to purification, p. 100.)

A great long-term advantage of purification is that our newly acquired senstivity will act like radar to screen out foods we formerly thought we had liked. It is amazing how we can become inured to foods that hurt us. But it is also amazing how a cleansed body can then instruct us intelligently.

Now for a warning: Purification is not a toy, not a gimmick. It involves serious, searching effort and can bring out deep reactions of the body-mind. Therefore it is highly advisable to become grounded in the daily practice of holistic nutrition before undertaking purification. *It is far more difficult to eat rationally on a daily basis than to restrict the diet radically.* Many people go on cycles of "purification" and random "binging" that are extremely detrimental to biological stability. They are not ready to purify.

Rejuvenation

Despite our general indifference to the natural, ongoing cellular process we call rejuvenation, our cells still replenish and regenerate. But what if we were aware of their beneficent role. What if we furthered it, appreciated it, enhanced it? We would indeed flourish!

Rejuvenation is a time — like purification — when our energy is *consciously* directed toward healing. It is a time of cellular meditation. It is a time for aware breathing and nutritional practices that will nurture cellular life. The diet consists of rejuvenatory catalysts, mineral-rich vegetables and herbs, and raw proteins appropriate for our situation.

In rejuvenation we are encouraging life, building life, and sharing life.

Sustenance

Sustenance is the biological process that empowers us to do our daily work. Simply put, it is our daily diet; but that does not tell the full story because the diet is the fuel for a nutritional process that must balance the demands of inner and outer forces on our being. It is a process that must afford a protective shield to guard against destructive agents in our daily life. The process must be attuned to our digestive capactiy and to our needs for protectioy, energy output, and rejuvenation.

The appropriate diet consists of whole grains, proteins, vegetables, fruit, and the various vitamins and herbs we have determined to be beneficial to our health.

As the song goes, "There is a time for everything under the sun," and so it is with the three modes of the nutritional process. There is a time for sustenance, for rejuvenation, for purification; and in the stage of stabilization we begin to sense these times and to orchestrate these modes in order to enhance our life. We will hear our body tapping out in a code, that only we know, its needs for rest and solitude, for play and intense activity, for nourishment, and for cleansing.

We will also begin to enhance these modes. For example, we can further purification by eating our last meal of the day earlier than six p.m. to provide about twelve hours for the digestive process — and if the last meal is light, so much the better. Another effective aid to purification is to eat lightly one day a week. Perhaps on your day of rest have a sabbath of the body too. Following the seasons dietarily also quickens purification. In the spring, when the cherries ripen, do some house cleaning!

There are also ways to encourage rejuvenation in our daily life. If we are attuned to our energy output, we know when we can eat lighter — perhaps totally of vegetables and light protein. Just so do we know when we need to eat protectively, appropriately to our flow of energy, to minimize the depletion of nutritional reserves and prevent illness; optionally, much of the time, sustenance is the emphasis.

External and Internal Ecology in Stabilization

As we can see from the discussion above of the three nutritional modes, the stabilized diet relates to not only ecology, our external environment, but to our inner ecology, our interior needs, and particularly (for our present purpose) to those needs that such factors as occupation, exercise, sex, love, sleep, climate and age bring into play.

So we need to take at least a brief look at how these factors fit in the stabilization stage.

Occupation – If your workplace has built-in stresses, whether from chemicals, noise, improper lighting (fluorescent light destroys vitamin C), or psychological pressures, the entire diet must focus on dealing with this challenge.

To begin with, it must contain suitable protein to deal with the corollary intestinal and digestive imbalances caused by stress; proper carbohydrates; high B-vitamin intake; and daily supplements of at least eight grams of vitamin C, 2400 I.U. of vitamin E, and minerals including balanced amounts of calcium, magnesium, and micro-doses of zinc and iodine.

As you can see, many occupations will have highly specialized needs.

Exercise – Optimal nutrition is simply not possible without the proper circulation of the blood that physical exertion stimulates. It is the distribution of nutrients through this circulation that enables the three modes of the nutritional process to operate.

Sex – If one engages in regular sexual activity that results in orgasm, it is wise to eat a diet rich in nucleic acids, proteins, and vegetables.

Love – If we can appreciate and nurture ourselves in ways that feed our body and soul and can receive love vibrations from those around us, then our ability to assimilate nutritional substances is greatly enhanced. If, on the other hand, we are negating our true self and are unable to receive love vibrations, our nutritional requirements increase because our assimilative functions will be impaired. We then need be more careful dietarily, concentrating on foods that will stabilize our blood sugar. Particularly whole grains, light proteins, gland-rebuilding herbs, and nutrients keyed to our uniqueness. See Chapter 7 on glands for additional help and also chapters on counseling, in particular, to promote the flow of love.

Sleep – Deep. peaceful sleep is a prerequisite for good health, for then — freed from the compulsions of our waking consciousness — our organism recharges and regenerates. It· is also a time when we may connect directly with our life spirit. It is a time to be enriched by dreams — if we but heed them.

Also, crucial reactions occur within the organism when we are resting. An entirely new group of hormones circulate to promote relaxation in order to meet the contingencies of the coming day.

Yet it is hardly a secret to point out that troubled sleep and sleeplessness are national complaints — in fact, that six out of ten people each night have difficulty sleeping. (You are not alone!) And no wonder: with our unnatural lifestyles, our chemicalized diet, and the extreme pressures of our intense culture.

Consequently, to meet such a condition dietarily requires a dramatic increase of the "light" proteins and an emphasis on vegetables, with an exclusion of such stimulants as salt, sugar, coffee, alcohol, etc., etc. It is also wise to utilize such herbs as chamomile, horsetail, oatstraw, and skullcap.

Deep breathing each day becomes essential through exercise or relaxation techniques since a lack of oxygen contributes to deep restlessness that prevents sleep. It is also important to sleep in a quiet, dark room (any light awakens sensors through the optic nerve).

It is also beneficial to keep the problems of the world out of your bed. Unload the problems of the day with someone beforehand, or else give yourself a counseling session. (See Chapter 2 for guidance.)

Climate – Weather and barometric conditions do affect our nutritional requirements. In warm weather we need more B vitamins (they are excreted through perspiration), and mineral-rich vegetables such as celery, parsley, zucchini, watercress.

In cold weather more fats, either animal or vegetable, and whole grains (to protect the vital sheath) are required.

Older persons – The dietary emphasis is on easily digestible foods that yield maximum assimilation. Such foods as light proteins (yogurt, egg yolk, raw milk, sprouted seed and nuts), fresh vegetable juices, steamed vegetables, and raw and stewed fruit are suggested — along with nutritional yeast and individually determined vitamin supplements.

Enzymes in Stabilization

We have already said that oxygenation is the key factor in nutrition. It stands to reason: without *consumed* oxygen we would not "burn" our food to obtain the energy necessary for life. Fortunately, this process of "ignition" has some doughty cohorts and facilitators in our enzyme system, for it is our enzymes that "work" the food in our system, that prepare the food for its literal consumption — which we call oxygenation.

But before we discuss enzymes further we need return briefly to underline the significance of oxygenation. A central fact highlights it: the brain uses twenty percent of our oxygen intake though it is only two percent of our body weight!

Actually all of the various rejuvenation programs have a common orientation of facilitating receptivity for those substances that transport oxygen to the cells. This is the potency of vitamin C, vitamin E, vitamin B15, gerovital and numerous "live-food" programs. An interesting footnote is that cancer can only survive in cells whose oxygen metabolism is abnormal.

Now you can see that though we are returning to a discussion of enzymes (for our sensitivity to them distinguishes this stage of our dietary transformation), how to eat, food harmonizations, intake-timing, food preparation practices, "power foods," and vitamins relate fundamentally to oxygenation — for that is the goal, the full transformation and utilization of our nutriment.

One further preliminary note. Some of the following considerations might seem remote. That is all right. What it probably implies is that more time need be spent in transition. However, bear in mind that the information is pertinent to the therapeutic application of nutrition.

When one eats aged, overcooked, and chemically induced and/or treated foods, it takes great enzymic capacity to digest them. They are a double jeopardy in that they do not contribute to their own digestion but must also draw on our enzyme reserves for their metabolism. A beautiful example of this may be seen in a contrast between raw and pasteurized milk: raw milk will naturally culture as it ages but pasteurized milk will putrefy. (Pasteurization destroys enzymes.)

Thus a daily pattern of eating beyond our enzymic capacity results in an impaired digestion that upsets assimilation and initiates metabolic disorder. Enzymic depletion is analogous to the feeling one gets after shopping all day during the holiday rush. It is the biological equivalent of being spent: no more juice to digest the juice.

Consequently food putrefies in our system, and it is putrefaction of proteins and the fermentation of carbohydrates within our body that create a state of toxemia which results in most of the common disorders of our time.

How To Eat in Stabilization

Eating is an exchange of energy, so it behooves you to know what you're exchanging. True, you're now learning about food. But did you know that the mood you are in when you eat is the mood you feed! That is why we must insure "eating readiness", for our external *and internal* world must be peaceful for proper nutrition.

If you are in a good mood and your "vibes" are harmonious, then digestion is greatly enhanced. Enzymes respond to emotion! If upset, it is better to sip cool water or go outside and breathe deeply before eating. A moment of silence and a prayer are the best appetizers. Or perhaps you need to talk to a friend "to get it out" — or else to your inner self, your inescapable best friend.

Chew your food well because your mouth is your first digestive organ, and it will veto the most thoughtful nutritional program if you are a fast eater. Yet we know how difficult it is to break that habit — after all, this whole, beautiful, crazy world we live in is based on speed.

That is why the prayer — or some other type of reflection — is helpful, for it sensitizes us for the exchange of energy by giving thanks to Mother Nature for her grace. You will also encourage proper chewing if you take a breath of air between mouthfuls. If you are one of those who naturally chew slowly and really enjoy their food, you are blessed!

Food Harmonization in Stabilization

(Every food is a note: make a good music!)

To eat well it is necessary to harmonize your food combinations, and yet never before have human beings been confronted with such a wide array of foodstuffs made available by a technology that can expedite their shipment from anywhere in the world or else create them (almost literally) in efficient food factories. This technology disturbs not only traditional food cultures all over the world but our own as well. Not only that, it upsets two beneficial "foodways" that personkind have long observed.

One way is to honor the produce of one's own climate and ecological environment, for — not so remarkably — *there* is the source of foods we most need. For food from our own environment is more vital to us since it contains just those substances we need to catalyze reactions that can deal with that environment. Another foodway now violated is the practice of eating seasonal foods.

But that wide array of food made available through technology exists, and needs to be confronted. Therefore the following remarks can be helpful in orchestrating our food choices in a harmonious way.

Proteins: These essential nutrients are best eaten at, or near, the beginning of a meal; the heavier proteins (cheese, meats, beans, amino-acid combinations) should be consumed at the beginning of the day. In nutritional therapy it is also important that only one concentrated protein be eaten at a meal. Proteins are best combined with vegetables, either raw or steamed. If you are in good health, they may be *satisfactorily* eaten with grains.

Vegetables: These are best eaten alone or with protein foods and grains. They are not happily mixed with fruit, though there are exceptions — notably the apple, papaya, pineapple, and banana.

Whole Grains: These energy foods are best with vegetables, sprouts, and dairy products. If you are in good health, they *can be* taken with seeds, nuts and other proteins. In nutritional therapy it is important not to eat sweets and grains. This combination, causing fermentation in the system, is a contributor to headache, eye tension, arthritis, and intestinal gas.

Fruit: These zestful foods are best eaten alone or between meals although they may also be eaten with yogurt or milk. The apple may be combined with vegetables or grain. Strong cleansing fruits such as grapes, cherries, melons, and citrus, should always be eaten alone. It is important *not* to eat fruit before meals. If you're upset, they'll cause an acidic reaction.

Liquids: Eat and drink separately. However a glass of fresh vegetable juice may be taken before eating for its digestive enzymes. If you feel thirsty after eating, it is a sign of too much salt or that the food was too concentrated (perhaps dried). Before resting for the night, it is often beneficial to have a sip of cool water.

Timing Your Meals

Although eating according to our energy expenditure and general vitality is a key principle for a balanced   nutritional   program, timing must correlate with intake or else the program will falter.

To begin our day, we insure the vital flow if we allow an hour or so after arising to intervene before eating. It is a time for being quiet, for being naked; for running and yoga; for listening and dancing to music. It is a time when, after rising, we need to wake up.

It is beneficial to sip some tea then from herbs you know to be congenial. (See the basic bruja tea recipe, p. 91.) Herbs are primitive, strong, majestic foods and the morning — when the world is being born — is an appropriate vibratory time to bathe the insides of our body with their healing essences. Then, after greeting the day with devotion, comes our nourishment.

What is eaten for breakfast must correlate with what you will do in the day. Breakfast is the most important meal of the day for your work performance; it is its nutritional foundation. It is then we provide ourselves with adequate sustenance, stabilizing blood sugar and insuring sufficient nucleic acids to nourish our cellular responses.

If you're going out into the world of automobile traffic, competitive vibrations and physical *or* mental labor, breakfast by all means should be substantial.

It should include whole grain, protein, perhaps fresh vegetable juice, nutritional yeast, and vitamin supplements. If your day will demand physical labor, then include more whole grain.

Nutritional intake the rest of the day will also be determined, of course, by energy requirements. If they will consist mainly of mental concentration, a diet of light protein, vegetables, and smaller amounts of grain is called for.

One of the most grievous dietary mistakes is the heavy dinner. This leads to indigestion, toxic bile, and the lack of appetite in the morning. When we are most exhausted, we eat the most. It makes no sense. It is then we need to relax, to replenish, to rejuvenate. Then, above all other time, do we need to feel just a little bit hungry when we leave the table. Remember: we will soon have some sleeping to do, some cellular regeneration to foster, and some dreams, perchance, to conduct.

Preparing Food

The way we prepare food reflects our attunement to its vital currents. If we think of it as a gift of life that possesses still many of the properties of life, we will respect its vitality in preparing it to replenish our own. Actually, when you have simplified your diet, food preparation will become amazingly easy.

The problem of course is that since most of the food we eat *is* lifeless, it can't be insulted further with torture-rack procedures (deep or heavy frying, insensitive boiling, destructive re-cooking, etc.), so that we form habits that are abhorrent to *live* food. We must protect the vital force in the food from the vital — but dangerous — force of fire. Unprotected, food is helpless before fire. Foods that are steamed or stewed slowly in water with low heat turn out best. A double boiler is a useful tool.

Two other "must" tools will also protect the life force in your food in order to assure maximum assimilation: First, is a hand grinder that can grind seeds and nuts into meal, and grains into cracked cereals and flour. What marvelous breakfast ingredients!

Next is a juicer — especially for fresh vegetable juices, which are assimilated in ten minutes and are the most enzyme-rich foods extant and so are prime nutritional candidates for rejuvenation programs (See Recipes for Meal No. 1, p. 97), nursing mothers, and those who do not, or cannot, eat vegetables.

Juices are also very helpful in stabilizing our nutritional program and are often essential in nutritional therapy.

Power Foods in Stabilization

As our diet becomes stabilized, we learn how to use "special foods." They are special not because they are exotic but because they are highly nutritious — yet often simple and commonly overlooked. They are special because they are powerful.

Nutritional Yeast – Yeast is a fantastic product! It is a single-cell protein living on such media as molasses, whey, and grain (some grow on wood chips and petroleum. but avoid them) and can be "farmed" with the most minimal resources; and yet it is the richest food source of the vitamin B complex and vegetable nucleic acids. It is a complete light protein, and it is indicated in all afflictions connected with blood-sugar metabolism and the nervous system. It is a lifeline for those used to "hanging on" to sugars and living under daily stress. It is very helpful in re-sensitizing the organism.

The best way to eat yeast is with enzyme-rich foods such as sprouts, vegetable juice, and yogurt or such fruit as apple and papaya. (mixed with ground seeds, oil and yogurt, it makes a marvelous salad dressing.)

All yeasts vary somewhat in nutritional components depending on what their growing medium is; therefore if you mix a few varieties, you'll get everything they offer. But even one variety is fine.

Baker's Yeast – Though it is more demanding to use, this *live* yeast is also a prime source of the B vitamins. It is also cheap and readily available. The difficulty is that you must eat it first thing in the morning with only water or milk and cannot eat other foods for at least thirty-five minutes on pain of disagreeable gas reactions.

Since it has a greater alkaline reaction than nutritional yeast, it can be safely used for an irritated intestine or colon and is very beneficial for ulcerated conditions. But once again: Use it carefully.

Sprouts — The richest source of essential rejuvenatory proteins and nucleic acids can be grown cheaply and easily in your own home!

The important sprouts are alfalfa, noted for its minerals; fenugreek, for its highly assimilable iron; lentils, for their nucleic acids; and sunflower seeds, for their protein, calcium, and vitamin B12.

When wheat is sprouted, it can be ground and baked for marvelous non-gluten-containing bread; or else the grass can be harvested and juiced.

Seaweed — The finest source of vegetable iron and iodine and all the known (and, very likely, many unknown) trace minerals, it has the power to draw poisons and chemicals out of the body into the intestines for elimination. It even offsets *some* of the effects of radiation.

It is an important and excellent addition to vegetable dishes and salads. It should be sprinkled on after cooking.

Homemade Yogurt — If it is homemade, it is highly useful for maintaining healthy intestinal flora; but remember that some storebought yogurt is so poorly produced it does not even contain friendly bacteria. In that case, one is better off just using straight acidophilus liquid or Eugalen Forte, a preparation of lactobacillus bifidus.

Algae — While not yet generally available, this single-cell protein will increasingly become an important survival food since it is rich in live proteins, nucleic acids, chlorophyll, and vitamin C.

In our lifetime we will see algae produced in every community, for it can be grown in fresh water by simply adding nutrients. First probably it will be introduced as an animal feed and as such will save an incredible amount of grain now fed to stock.

This is an all-round power food, and when people will get over its novelty and its distinctive taste, they will prize its precious qualities.

Herbs — It is not the province of this book to go into detail on this subject, but we must say enough to get you started with nature's most complete and precise healing food and medicine.*

First, they must be respected in order to work. You must attune to the water they brew in and to its interaction with plant and fire for a medicinal transfer of energy within your blood.

Now here is a basic bruja herbal mixture. It is just one example of a multitude of nutritious combinations of herbs that you can prepare and use daily. First boil the five roots for twelve minutes and then steep the other herbs for twenty-four minutes.

Roots (boil for 12 minutes)

licorice — For the lungs and endocrine system (1/4 measurement)
dandelion — For the liver
burdock — Also for the liver
comfrey root — For the lungs (purifies the blood)
angelica — For the etheric body (1/6 measurement)

Stems and Flowers (steep for 24 minutes)

comfrey — Rich in minerals, synthesizes vitimin B12
nettles — Extremely rich in minerals, especially organic sodium
horsetail — Rich in silicon, which transmutes to calcium
peppermint — A digestive-enzyme enhancer
chamomile — A specific for colds and flu; calcium-rich, soothing
alfalfa — Rich in minerals and vitamins A and K, also pyridoxine
cleavers — For the kidney and bladder

* A good recourse for further information is the California School of Herbal Studies, P.O.Box 350, Guerneville, Ca. 95446

VITAMINS

Basic Daily Maintenance Vitamin Program

Of course, the best way to get one's vitamins is through our food, as most of the medical profession claim does happen. But unfortunately, as even more of that same profession are beginning to recognize, that is not the case. Our food — unless it is carefully and organically grown — is now sadly deficient.

It should be borne in mind that the following treatment of vitamins is a general guide to daily maintenance and is intended to supplement a diet that is well into the transition and has not been modified to deal with special disturbances. In any case, if you feel a vitamin program would be of benefit to you, we suggest you obtain professional advice for your special individual needs.

Actually, for many heavy vitamin supplementation is not appropriate. Since, at least in naturopathic therapy, the cause of physiological impairment is seen to be a depletion of vital force, it is by no means certain that energy imbalance can be laid at the doorstep of vitamin deficiency. But *in most cases* there are sufficient nutritional side effects from imbalance to make vitamin *therapy* very rewarding.

The following, then, are brief descriptions of some of the vitamins that may aid us in our nutritional transformation.

Vitamin C — Vitamin C is found in living foods, fresh foods. It is the freshness factor and it keeps us fresh. It keeps us fresh by bringing oxygen into our cells. It keeps us fresh by catalyzing a myriad of vital processes — such as the transport of iron in red blood cells and the support of our defensive forces for daily detoxification.

For city dwellers it is wise to use anywhere from two to eight grams daily, the dosage depending on the extent and intensity of stress. For days with exhaust fumes, tobacco smoke, fluorescent light, air conditioning and gas heat — or with psychological pressure — eight grams is not too much.

The most advantageous way to use supplemental C is to take it at mealtime *with* foods containing this magic cleanser and elixir. We recommend vitamin C with Meal Number 1 (see recipes), fresh fruit, sprouts, fresh vegetable juice, etc.

Vitamin E – This vitamin is found in foods containing strong regenerative powers. Seed power. It increases our stamina and strength by getting oxygen to the red blood cells, so that it is a marvelous handmaiden to the heart and lungs.

Vitamin E should be naturally derived, and taken at the end of a meal consisting of some oils or fat or foods rich in the vitamin, since it is *only fat-soluble*.

Daily dosage will again depend on the relative stress of your daily life. However, at least 2,400 I.U. from mixed tocopherols are advised daily. For therapeutic usage one should combine the mixed and the D alpha tocopherols.

Foods rich in this adrenal-gland healer are egg yolks, seeds and nuts, vegetable oils, avocado, wheat germ, sprouted wheat bread, carrot juice, and nettles.

Vitamin B Complex — Here is a significant stress vitamin especially fortifying for contemporary nervous systems, which must receive, compute, and program an incredible amount of input from this "power-grid world." As its increasing demands impinge on our skins and nerves, so does the need of this complex increase exponentially.

Like vitamin C this group of vitamins is water soluble and so can penetrate into every cell of the body. They flow with water, they are light, and they have to do with responses that move like light within the entire nervous system. They are a supreme nerve food.

Some — like B6 — work through the adrenal glands to stimulate secretions of optimism; some — like niacin and B1 — are specifics for depression and anxiety; others — like B15 and folic acid — help oxygenate the red blood cells; and still another vitamin, B17, helps maintain proper sugar metabolism, thereby starving cancer cells.

It is so difficult to discuss the role of vitamins without relating them to the *networks* of relationships that they influence. For example, sulphur, essential to body tissues and proper digestion, is also needed for the synthesis of vitimin B1.

Also our B-vitamin balance crucially affects the thyroid — which in turn is affected by blood sugar levels. And when the liver is impaired, our entire B-vitamin balance will be skewed so that we need make corrections with sensitive use of B-vitamin-rich foods.

Furthermore, if the B-vitamins are not adequately supported with such minerals as molybdenum, copper, and magnesium (vital to the transport and synthesis of hemoglobin) they will not facilitate the catalytic messages these micro-nutrients must convey to the brain.

B-vitamin supplements need be taken with meals containing such B-vitamin-rich foods as nutritional yeast, whole grain, yogurt, seeds and nuts, liver, miso, and eggs. It is important to get a formula with balanced constituents.

Vitamin A – Since vitamin A promotes cellular growth and repair and fights infection, it is often suggested for nourishing the tiny lung cells affected in bronchitis, asthma, and pneumonia. Vitamin A is also valuable for liver impairment from alcohol, hepatitis, or sugar addiction; however it is then necessary to obtain the vitamin from both animal and vegetable sources since an impaired liver cannot synthesize the vitamin-A-bearing carotene.

The supplement should be taken with such foods rich in this vitamin as egg yolk, liver, winter squash, carrots, sweet potatoes, turnip greens, parsley, persimmons, apricots, lemon grass, and dandelion greens.

Most vitamin-A preparations are made from fish liver oils, but there is also a vegetarian product from lemon grass and other herbs. It is important that this vitamin be fresh. Oils do go rancid.

A basic daily recommended dosage would be 25,000 units — after meals containing oils. There has been a great scare about vitamin A toxicity. This can happen, to be sure, through reckless pill-popping or chomping polar bear liver, but it is a highly improbable danger.

Vitamin D – The sunshine vitamin. The sun's rays meet the living skin and a process is initiated that metabolizes this vitamin.

The best time for hunting and gathering this vitamin is mornings, when the sun's ultra-violet light is most absorbable; an adequate supply is important since, for one thing, it promotes the proper absorption of calcium and phosphorus.

Fine sources are egg yolks, fish liver oils, sunflower seeds, shitake mushrooms, nettles, and milk (especially in the summer).

CONCLUSION

Here we are at the end of our nutritional journey . . . Or is it the end of the beginning? Frankly, we hope it is. We sincerely hope that you will go back now, if you need to, and truly experience — slowly, at your own pace — the awareness, the transition, and the stabilization stages in order to feel the connection that we opened the chapter with — the connection that nutrition can make with breath and life, with peace, and with the psyche.

We hope that as you purify, rejuvenate, and sustain yourself you will move to an ecological consciousness of a new age. All of us desperately need to see through the facades of the dying order the radiant sun of our new being.

What is so wonderful about the nutritional process is that all of us — through our nature — are a part of it and so have the power — through awarenss — to awaken to not only what is essential for our own well-being but also for the continuation of life on the planet.

Nutrition is a science that can only be truly appreciated by those who can *participate* in the vitality of nature for themselves and others. As such it is truly a human science, and it is fast becoming recognized as perhaps the most potent tool for offsetting the terrible spread of degenerative disease.

We hope that this journey will have helped you to be open not only to food but, more importantly, to the natural you, the you that hungers for a better life and is ready to journey toward it.

Recipes

Recipes for Optimal Health
"the kind the people eat"

When, as a child, I would ask my father what we were going to have for breakfast, he used to say "the kind the people eat." I now know what he meant, and I appreciate him for connecting my food to the food of people all over the globe.

Actually, what we eat for breakfast and the other meals of our day is very related to who we become in that day. To be in new ways we need to eat in new ways — in ways that express our unique place in the universe. We can eat in ways that honor the earth and respect ourselves.

The most difficult aspect of eating is being in touch with what we need. If we would just *listen* to our needs, eating would become a constantly interesting experience.

The following recipes are just suggestions. They are examples of food harmonizations. Of course, one does not need recipes to attune to food. One needs respect. When I was seventeen, I co-founded the first vegetarian restaurant in Berkeley, California. I had never read a recipe, nor had I ever cooked for the public; but I did have a profound respect for the vital force in food. Apparently this respect carried over into the preparations because our patrons enjoyed their meals.The restaurant is still serving heathful foods to the public.

Recipes must also be appropriate to one's life. When healthy we eat differently than when sick. When active we eat differently than when at rest. Therefore, I have divided these recipes into the following categories: Eating for work, Eating light, and Fasting.

Eating for Work

Generally, when we are active and working, we need two meals a day that contain complete protein and are rich in nucleic acids, vitamins, and minerals. The following are examples of such meals. The amount to be used depends on your appetite.

1. Meal Number One: This meal is not only good for work, it is excellent for rejuvenation. It is truly one of the most beneficial meals I have experienced.

    To begin with, make yourself a glass of juice from carrot, apple, and one, or more, of the following greens — parsley, celery, spinach, etc. Pour juice in a bowl and add:
    yogurt
    sprouts (either alfalfa, fenugreek, sunflower, or lentil)
    almonds (ground)
    nutritional yeast
    ground seeds (sunflower, pumpkin, and chia)
    chopped apple, sliced banana, or cooked millet or oats may also be added to the basic ingredients.

2. Whole Grain Combination: To a mixture of cooked millet, buckwheat, and brown rice, add:
    ground seeds and nuts
    sprouts
    This basic mixture may be eaten with either milk, honey, and apple or oil, seaweed, and soy sauce.

3. Steamed Vegetables: Steam string beans, zucchini, celery root, winter squash, jerusalem artichokes (and/or any of *your* favorites).
    To this basic mixture add;
    sprouts
    whole grain
    ground seeds and nuts or two egg yolks
    garlic, rosemary, parsley, celery

4. Salad: Grate raw beets and carrots and mix with spinach, sprouts, and celery. Ground seeds and nuts may be added to the raw vegetables as well as garlic, olive oil and lemon, to flavor.

5. Real Cereal
    A. granola style:
        2 cups oatmeal
        ½ cup   nutritional yeast
        ¼ cup honey (optional)
        2 cups (combined) of ground corn, rice, and millet
        1 tbs. kelp powder
        Ingredients are spread thinly on a baking sheet and baked slowly until toasted lightly. Ground sunflower, sesame, almonds, and pumpkin seeds may be added after baking.
    B. peasant style:
        Place coarse-ground brown rice, corn, millet, oats, buckwheat, and rye in a double boiler or saucepan and cook very slowly for an hour.

6. Sunflower - sprout cheese:
    Place sprouted sunflower seeds in a blender and blend with sesame oil, garlic, and kelp. This mixture may then be spread on sprouted wheat bread, eaten with raw or steamed vegetables, or eaten alone.

7. Tofuna:
   Place tofu in mixing bowl and add:
   >   celery
   >   onions
   >   chopped parsley
   >   soy sauce
   >   oil
   This mixture may be eaten with salad and/or grain.

8. Far-out Mung Sprout:
   Steam your favorite vegetables and then add:
   >   mung sprouts
   >   garlic
   >   rye sprouts
   >   celery
   To this mixture may be added seeds or nuts. It may be eaten with whole grain combinations or salad.

Eating Light

Some days, when we have the space, it is very beneficial to eat light. The following are suggestions for light meals:
1. juice of carrot, apple, and some greens
2. mix carrot juice with fresh milk and a half papaya
3. two raw eggs blended with milk and honey
4. fresh fruit in season
5. yogurt, fresh fruit, nutritional yeast, and sprouts
6. goat milk with herbal tea
7. brown rice, apples or apple sauce, and milk
8. millet, alfalfa sprouts, and sesame oil.
9. fresh apple juice with yogurt and nutritional yeast
10. oatmeal, kudzu (a marvelous root!), and apples

Fasting

Purification should always be entered into with care and perspective. For example, there are some disorders — such as hepatitis and cancer — that call for purification, but in a special regimen.

Fasting Combinations
1. Sodium and Potassium Broth:
    Steam zucchini, parsley, celery, and string beans. These vegetables may be eaten whole, or blended in a broth.
2. Fruit Juice Blend:
    To the juice of fresh apple, grape, and grapefruit add blended whole papaya and pineapple. This juice can be diluted with distilled water. It is excellent for an over-proteinized condition.
3. Carrot, apple, parsley, and celery juice.
4. A blend of goat milk, alfalfa sprouts, and apple juice.
5. A juice blend of fresh comfrey leaves, borage, parsley, lettuce, and apples.
6. Combine raw goat's milk with the tea of fenugreek seed, cascara bark, alfalfa, caraway seed, and peppermint. Excellent for sugar addiction.
7. Mix lemon, lime, and water. May be taken with vitamin C.
8. Fresh fruit in season, one to a meal (grapes, cherries, persimmons, figs, apricots, apples, peaches, plums, watermelon, etc.)
9. Santa Rose Hips: apple juice with rose hip powder and honey.
10. Live yeast and milk.
11. Water

The Endocrines:

DESTINY OR DELIVERANCE

For at least 1,500 years it used to be thought in the Western world that both the personality and the physical type of people were largely determined by their glands. From the Middle Ages through the Eighteenth Century at least, the general theory was that the mixture and proportions of a person's "humours" (there were four: blood, phlegm, yellow bile, and black bile) were the main determinants.

In the Nineteenth Century physiologists learned much more precise information about glands and the entire endocrine system and the effects of their functions or malfunctions — so that human beings became in their eyes even more the products of uncontrollable internal mechanisms. You were a particular type — whether thyroid, pituitary, or adrenal — and there was little you could do about it but make the best of it, although eventually they learned how to operate and to inject secretions.

This inescapable logic of the glands, this concept of being trapped by one's physiology, finally lost its authority somewhere in the 'Twenties when the message of modern psychology began to be heard to the effect that we were far more the victims of our subjective history — but that we could do something about that: we could liberate ourselves from it through the power of consciousness.

People naturally breathed a sigh of relief, and so they began to be psychoanalyzed, and later, self-actualized as they embraced the humanistic tenets of contemporary psychology. Many decided they could, by and large, control their personal destiny — if not their collective history. They could insure their own liberation. Glands were relegated to medical specialists and to the operating room.

We believe that this was an advance, that people in large degree can master their fate, but not by ignoring their internal system of homeostasis, largely governed by their glandular and endocrine system. We believe it is necessary to *understand* our glandular inheritance — its advantages, its potential, its style of integrating reality, its "signature"; but also its biases, its pitfalls, its dangerous proclivities — in order to truly master fate, for ignorance is not mastery but delusion.

And the reality is that our physical organism does correlate with psychological functions: our emotions and feelings are related to the physical body. The principle of ecology is just as applicable to our Being (the body-mind-spirit) as to the earth that nourishes us. In fact we call the ways in which our physical make-up and our psychological behavior correlate "lines of interaction." Where we differ from previous gland specialists is that we say: our bodies are not only our destinies, they are also our deliverance!

Awareness

The secret is in awareness. One line of interaction is our digestive, assimilative, and eliminative functions. Another is our manifold glandular system. But remember: both translate into a behavioral language that we can "read" — and thus honor, moderate, or contradict.

It's true that what we receive from the external environment is determined by our social and genetic history — but only in part! We also have judgment, which can choose what we want to interact with and what we want to get out of it. Once again: the way out of glandular destiny is the realization that since glands affect consciousness, consciousness affects glands. It is possible to orchestrate our bio-psychological behavior by honoring our uniqueness and offsetting the deficits.

Only by being aware of our individual lines of interaction can we transcend them to become a more well-rounded person through the application of nutritional, bio-elemental, and psychological practices. After all, we cannot even be sure what is inherited and what congenital. Many environmental factors influence our legacy: the way we were born, the quality of milk we were fed, the familial vibrations we became conditioned to, and the socio-political ways in which we were programed to express ourselves.

The latter is very important since a sexist society chooses for us the line of interaction that is most appropriate to the sexual role we have been born to play — regardless of our unique inherited glandular "geography." For example, the male is often induced to co-opt the adrenal function (the effects of the functions of our glands on our personalities will be explained shortly), whereas the female manifests herself thyroidally. As if the glands recognize these sex-role patterns of behavior that so distort the human bio-psyche!

So the beginning of work in this realm is learning to say no to this kind of exploitation of our own energy. This respect can be a first step in aligning ourselves with forces that can make the world responsive to the real needs of human beings rather than to the fragmenting competitive demands of social systems.

After all, our health is determined by the way we take in our external environment: in large chunks of food, in vibrations and impressions, and in water, air, and light. Our ability to digest what we ingest, assimilate what we experience, and eliminate the residues of these processes *is* our life.

This natural functioning we call life is maintained by an array of organs and glands designed by nature to maintain homeostasis. These organs and glands function most efficiently, of course, with an optimal load. Yet a conditioned disregard of our unique energy flow will raise the load and so impair our naturally designed organs of digestion, assimilation, and elimination. We lose the ability to be in the present.

We typically cause this impairment by eating unawarely to re-establish a homeostasis upset by a discordant physical and emotional "diet". Rather than change our environment and/or discharge our feelings we overeat or eat badly — so that eventually our digestive enzymes are depleted (very likely from overcooked proteins and lifeless food) and our stomach and bowels are inflamed with acidic indigestion and irritating fecal matter.

The Liver

When our kidneys become clogged with the acids of coffee, drugs, protein indigestion, etc., our system must seek help to metabolize the overload in our blood; and so it inevitably calls upon a most complex and miraculous organ to remedy the imbalance — the liver.

Actually the liver is our largest endocrine gland: its functions are incredibly vast and varied*. It both acts as an intermediary between our digestive and glandular functions and converts the amino acids we eat to our own unique protein configurations, as well as neutralizing and eliminating poisons, drugs, and excessive hormone accumulation from the system. It accomplishes the latter through the excretory secretion of bile.

The liver also prepares foods for oxidation, stores surplus nourishment for future use, and is involved in the digestion of fats and the maintenance of the blood sugar level.

So the proper functioning of the liver is of utmost importance to good health. However, when it begins to fail as a blood filter, toxic substances inevitably enter the general blood circulation, initiating the first phase of a highly significant — and generally misunderstood — abnormal process of homeostasis that naturopathic medicine calls "vicarious elimination." It is vicarious because the liver must then "choose' other endocrine systems (and they in turn call other organ systems) to do the unfinished work.

Now is where the process gets complicated. Not only relative to the endrocrine system chosen (which we will go into in detail) but to the manifold diseases that occur when these toxic substances invade unfamiliar channels, areas, and organs unequipped to handle the deadly onrush (most doctors prescribe for the symptoms precipitated by the invasion rather than confronting the patient's lifestyle and its main consequence, liver fatigue.).

But to return to the question of the endocrine system chosen once the liver must default, it is necessary to recall that sexual roles determined by social conditioning play a large part here, along with, of course, genetic propensities.

---

*typologies in this chapter are based on the pioneering research of Dr. Henry Bieler, M.D. We refer you to his book "Food is Your Best Medicine".

Since most individuals genetically acquire a tendency toward one of three glandular typologies, it will be useful to describe them before going on to our methology of balance through nutritional, bio-elemental, and psychological practices.

Adrenal Gland

First the adrenal glands, which direct elimination through the kidneys and bowels. Located near, and participating with, the kidneys in a symbiotic relationship, they are generally opted for as the masculine system by males since the adrenals function by powering through things and since technological life demands a driving energy from the adrenals to cope with the stresses of danger, noise, and smell.

Of course, since man was hunter, they have been drawn on as a masculine resource — and still are in the competitive business world, so that naturally or by role compulsion men generally function as dominant "adrenaloids," or else they feel inadequate and/or crazy. Of course some choose "feminine" lifestyles. There is also another possibility: They can become aware of the distortions and absurdity of sexual roles and then choose their own path ! They can regain the ability to nurture and be sensitive to the more subtle experiences and vibrations of life...

Thyroid Gland

The thyroid, located in the throat, responds to emergencies by directing elimination through the various layers of skin and the mucous and serous membranes. Since it influences the rate of perception of feelings, it is associated with a feminine mode of behavior and so opted for by females regardless of their natural bent — unless of course they have been liberated in the feminist awakening.

The thyroid secretes the feminine equivalent of sperm into every blood cell that passes through it in the form of an iodine compound.

The thyroid-dominant individual acutely senses not only the outside world but engages as well in an ongoing internal dialogue so that there are usually two simultaneous mental currents operative. For this reason, "thyroids" must become attuned to expressing sensitivity. The imbalanced thyroid function is either manifested in overly dramatic or repressed emotional behavior.

Pituitary Gland

Finally, the pituitary, located at the base of the brain — called our master gland because it gears with potentiality, power, primal force, and the integration of all sexuality. Its energy is symbolized by unity. It is the unified flowing energy in our veins and meridians, arteries and chakras. It is directly responsive to the functioning of the other endocrines.

Pituitary-dominant persons are associated with creative energy, sexual expression, mentation, and dreaming. The ways they manifest their intuitional and primal force determine the balance they strike between their own demands and those of the world. When they live in conflict with their basic natures, they arouse a wide range of biochemical reactions that inevitably trigger the pituitary itself into intense activity.

Working Together

Unfortunately, though individual descriptions of glands are necessary, they tend to give the impression of independent functioning; and yet all the glands are totally interconnected. Their separation is purely linguistic!

For example, when the metabolism is low, the level of thyroid hormone in the blood must rise. But since the blood flow during thyroid secretion is heavier in that gland than in other parts of the body, the pituitary produces a thyroid stimulant to right the balance. Furthermore, the pituitary has a direct relationship with the adrenals since it controls the secretion of corticoids that adjust the storage of glycogen in the liver.

The glands too underline the Great Lesson — we are all one . . .

Self Attunement

The following exercises are designed for self-attunement to our basic energy flow. The processes they initiate will enable you to discover the ways you use your energy and methods for balancing it. From these processes, then, you can continue the "Work" in a systematic and intelligible way.

First it would be helpful to read all three glandular typologies to find the one that fits you and then to pursue the pertinent exercises.

Please remember that the three typologies are not exclusive. We all have characteristics in all the typologies. That is the beauty of the human: we are all expressions of the One. We transform energy in unique ways, but we all transform the same energy through very similar bodies.

The main point is that by discovering how we transform energy we can be better able to master its changes, better able to honor our unique ways of transformation.

In the exercises you will be asked to visualize various colors in the bio-elemental work. Many have a profound effect on our being: some are invigorating (toning); and other are soothing (calming). The color you choose to visualize will be determined by the effect you need.

The four elements may also be used for these "special effects," as indicated in the exercises. For example, if water is suggested, you may bathe or swim in it, run alongside it, meditate on it, etc. If air is indicated, you may, of course, breathe awarely or bathe in it or meditate on it or perhaps think of how you can air out your life, etc.

Enjoy your work. It is beneficial — and revealing.

I.   *Adrenal Glands* — third chakratic sphere*
      Our "Solar Plexus Force"
      They actualize by "doing it!"
      • *Adrenal function* is associated with: the regulation and
        control of nervous energy.
      • general physical energy and internal generation of heat
      • control of voluntary and involuntary muscles
      • blood pressure, circulation
      • body immunity
      • secretions of anti-inflammatory hormones
      • oxidation of all body tissues

Physical Characteristics of the Typical Adrenal-Dominant Person:

Hair: of head, course, often curly; body hair, thick

Eyes: dark blue, brown or black

Forehead: low, often with low hairline

Nose: well developed, with large nostrils

Teeth: large, resistant to caries

Lips: full, with strong ruddy color

Skull: wide across temples, lower jaw heavy and often protruding

Ears: lobe thick, large and long

Chest: broad; heart and lungs large

Abdomen: wide, often protuberant

Extremities: thick and short

Genitals: large

Skin: thick, dry, warm

Profile: "Adrenals" have great energy and need physical exertion to
express it. They are basically optimistic. They trust themselves and
others. They have strong digestive and eliminative powers. They
are generally easygoing and sleep deeply and well (so well they
usually do not remember dreams).

---

*"Chakra" is a medical term from an ancient Indian Aruvedic system of esoteric
physiology. It is still used by many — in acupuncture, yoga, and other Eastern
systems. The term is used here only for such practitioners. The following exercises
are perfectly usable without additional information.

They are often unaffected by the surrounding "vibes". They feel good and they like to work, play, eat big meals, and enjoy. Since their sexual drive is strong, they find it very difficult not to engage in regular sexual relations. Their stamina is excellent.

With strong digestive abilities, they have an inclination to over-eat, especially sweet starches. This leads to sluggishness that is often compensated for with such adrenal stimulants as salt, coffee, chocolate and meat.

Adrenals, unless they know the "Work", run excessively on adrenal energy and gradually become exhausted. The fine attri-butes of their physical body — their strength and end-urance — become their undoing.

Eliminative Channels: Since adrenals can store large amounts of toxins in the lymph system, they are not often sick; but when they are it is often a serious healing crisis. When the adrenals become exhausted, they may activite the kidneys into "vicarious" elimina-tion, and both may "borrow" oxidizing power from the other. When adrenals and kidneys become depleted, then the lungs are the next organs of vicarious elimination — and sometimes the ears. The adrenal person also eliminates heavily through the bow-els.

The Work: Adrenals need to know they are all right in themselves — even when "not doing". They need to accept feel-ing good and deserving love for just being. It is useful for them to become more sensitive to their environment and their own inner feelings, and to the feelings of those around them. They also must develop "integral power" rather than induced stimulation; there-fore clarification of goals becomes essential.

Nutritional Needs: A basic wholesome diet should emphasize ample whole grains (to conserve protein and provide blood sugar stability) and raw vegetable juices and salads as well as steamed vegetables. Rich in vitamin A and E and the phospholecithins, wheat germ oil and raw egg yolks are specific rejuvenation foods for the adrenals. It is essential that the adrenal person not eat meat in excess. Raw seeds and nuts can provide excellent protein.

Mineral Requirements and Herbal Sources

calcium — oat straw, chamomile
chlorine — celery, parsley
iron — burdock root, fenugreek seed
silicon — horsetail
phosphorus — caraway seed, licorice
sulphur — nettles, garlic
manganese — wintergreen, mushrooms

Bio-elemental Work: (Symbolized by the element fire and the color scarlet) Adrenals are calmed by the element water and the color purple. Air and magenta are their toning agents.

Cellular Meditation for the Adrenals: Inhale through nose and out the mouth, letting the jaw drop and articulating on the exhale, "Ahhhhhhhh."
Breathe gently — evenly, fully.
As you inhale, breathe in the Life Force.
Feel this force circulate throughout your entire being.
Feel this force, knowing that it is the emanation of the One Great Spirit.
Now, relax your chest as you exhale completely.
Feel your openness.
Feel the vibrating current of the life force in your aura.
Feel your body as the residence of your soul.
Feel your connection with all life. Radiate peace.
Now breathe in and out the nose — gently, evenly and fully.
Breathe in the life force imbued with your desired color. (See above.)
Breathe in the soles of your feet (as if your feet could breathe) and slowly bring your breath up your legs, relaxing every part of your body before moving on.
Now focus on exhaling slowly and completely, letting go of anything you need to let go of. Then again inhale through the soles of your feet, feeling a circle of energy.
Now feel the circle completing its path: your own wholeness! You can enjoy just feeling your wholeness, your Essential Being.

II. *Thyroid Glands* — fifth chakratic sphere —
Our expressive force.

Thyroid function is associated with:

- sugar liberation from the liver to the bloodstream
- the heart beat
- acute sensory perceptions
- rate of metabolism
- expression of movement
- thyroxin — the "wake-up" secretion

The Thyroid controls the rate of metabolism: the rate at which we exchange ourselves with the world. The Thyroid function greatly increases during any toxic condition.

Physical characteristics:

Hair: (of head) fine and silky; body hair, thin, finely distributed

Features: delicate, finely molded

Eyes: large

Teeth: large, narrowly spaced, prone to decay

Tongue: moderately thin, long

Neck: graceful and long

Chest: long, with thin, sensitive nipples

Abdomen: long

Genitals: medium-sized (sensitive)

Extremities: finely moulded; neither stubby nor markedly elongated.

Profile: Thyroidals are sensitive. They can be acutely vulnerable to "vibes" — to environmental conditions and interpersonal relations. Their own highly sensitive projections often distort other people's meanings. Their concentration is often divided by two concurrent trains of thought. Their internal secretions (from the liver, kidneys, salivary glands) are highly active.

The Work: Thyroidal individuals generally need to learn to feel without taking everything personally. They need to "own" the nurturing quality of their interactions but also to be aware of their exhausting nature; and it is helpful for them to learn to express themselves in ways that both honor their feelings and respect those of other people. They often require more sleep and "alone time" than others. Calm, thoughtful people in peaceful surroundings contribute to their balance. Periods of sexual abstinence to utilize sexual energy for self-healing are very helpful. If thyroidals do not attune to their heightened sensitivity, they may close off from the world, slowing down and getting fat.

Nutritional needs: Because the rate of metabolism may oscillate between rapid and sluggish, it is advisable for thyroidals to attune to their digestive powers. The solution is often smaller and more frequent meals. Special foods include seaweed, vital uncooked proteins and sprouted wheat, the calcium-rich stems of plants, and sunflower and sesame seeds.

Mineral Requirements and Herbal Sources:
iodine — seaweed, dulce, garlic
calcium — chamomile, oatstraw, horsetail
magnesium — mullein, alfalfa, corn silk
chlorine — celery, fennel, nettles
potassium — borage, comfrey root, yarrow
sodium — anise, nettles, celery

Eliminative Channels: Thyroid gland directs elimination through the three layers of skin:

Inner skin: body linings (excess elimination causes bronchitis, appendicitis)
Middle skin: joints (excess causes arthritis, bursitis, neuritis)
Outer skin: hide (excess causes eczema, psoriasis)

Bio-elemental work: (symbolized by the "fifth element" ether and the color blue).

The thyroid is calmed by the element water and the color indigo. Fire (watching, meditating on; the breathing exercise, "breath of fire"; the sun) is the toning agent for the thyroid, as is the color golden orange.

Cellular Meditation:

Inhale through the nose and exhale through the mouth (completely breathing) gently, evenly, fully.
Feel your entire being filling with vital force.
Now as you inhale, imagine a candle in your solar plexus and then light it...
As you continue breathing:
Feel the warmth radiate upward to your heart.
Feel your lungs receiving life.
Feel your chest expand and open.
Feel the life force within.

Next, inhaling through the nose and exhaling through the nose, inhale as you imagine you are bringing the breath up through the soles of your feet — gently, evenly, fully — to your throat area. Feel the vital current circulate and nourish.
Exhale completely, feeling your healing energy vitalized by the love in your heart. Sense the miracle of creation within you. Swim in the ocean of serenity.

Now, as you breathe, become conscious of the warmth in your solar plexus area, and with the awareness of this center initiate a current of energy from the plexus to the thyroid body, sending the warm solar plexus energy along in your channel.
Having generated your current, now take your right hand and gently place it on your thyroid gland and gently "milk" this area:
Feel the healing secretions forming, feel the hormone of tranquillity balancing your sensitivity, feel your true strength and the Essence of your Being in the center of creation.

III. Pituitary - seventh chakratic sphere —
Our force for union and harmony.

The pituitary has been thought of as the master gland, though current research seems to be indicating that the pineal body and other parts of the brain may soon share this distinction. In any case, the pituitary is profoundly important.

Pituitary function:
- associated with seven vital hormones, most of which activate other endocrines
- circulation of fluids and water metabolism
- body temperature and fat metabolism
- the sexual control center

The pituitary is like the liver. It functions as the intermediary betwen the other endocrine glands and the entire organism. Its principal function is balancing, the creation of an integral harmony.

Physical characteristics:

Head: large; skull high, often dome-like, frontal bone and superior orbital ridges often prominent
Features: long upper lip
Teeth: usually large
Joints: unusual laxity; knock-knees, flat feet common
Extremities: legs and arms long; fingers long and thin

Profile: Pituitary-dominant persons are driven by a creative urge. There is often an artistic inclination, but this may be sublimated by daydreaming, fantasy life, and sexual preoccupation. There is a need for deep emotional content in their lives, and if this is lacking, they often form sentimental attachment to the past.

Eliminative Channels: Pituitary-dominants will often vicariously eliminate through either the pituitary itself— causing swelling and headaches — or through the sexual organs. In the male this organ would be the prostate gland; in the female, the uterus. They also may use sex to relieve themselves of psychic tension and blood toxicity.

Very sensitive to salts of all kinds, they nevertheless — more than most people — can absorb their toxic properties into the cerebrospinal fluid, which circulates to the brain.

The Work: The most difficult task for "pituitaries" is to emerge from their person dramas and their superiority complexes to consolidate unity with others. Although this conflict may seem paradoxical since the pituitary gland furthers balance, their egos often stand in the way. But those pituitaries who overcome their exploitive natures will be possessed with incredible energy. By the same token, they must re-examine their sexual life so that it will also express their love. Otherwise they will be enmeshed in all the karma of superficial sexual gratification.

Nutritional Needs: The diet indicated is one grounded in whole foods with an emphasis on mineral-rich vegetables, herbs and "light" proteins. Essential for maintaining biochemical stability is the elimination of all artificial foods and drugs which pituitaries often crave. Indeed, they are especially prone to depression and excitement associated with drug use. The sugar-starch combination (forming alcohol in the system) is particularly damaging to them.

Mineral Requirements and Herbal Sources
manganese — strawberry leaves, peppermint, mushrooms
sulphur —nettles, garlic, raw cabbage
phosphorus —chickweed, caraway seed, licorice
iodine — fo-ti-teng (Chinese herb), Irish moss

Bio-elemental work: (Symbolized by the element
air and the color indigo)
The pituitary is calmed by the element water
and the color turquoise. It is toned by the element
earth and the color green.

Cellular Meditation: Breathe through the nose
and out the mouth, feel your physical body eas-
ing.
Imagine you are lying on sand.
Feel your body giving in to the sand.
You are in your body . . .
Surrender . . . surrender.
Surrender to your own realness, your own
inherent vitality.
You are in your body.
It is the inside of the One.
Now, breathing through the nose and exhaling
from the nose, breathe slowly, gently, evenly.
As you inhale, breathe in the soles of your
feet.
Really appreciate your feet as the part of you
that embrace the earth constantly.
Feel the connection between your feet and
your head as you breathe, and bring the
breathe up from your feet to your head.
Appreciate the unity of You as you breathe.
Now, as your breath reaches your sacrum (base of
the spine), focus on the apex of this sacred
triangle and begin to follow your vital current up
your spinal cord.
Actually get inside your spinal cord and flow
upward with the cerebrospinal fluid. Then
concentrate on your third eye, exhaling out
the top of your head.
Finally, make a circuit: inhale through the feet,
raise the breath throughout the organism, and

then exhale out the top of the head, feeling the
circle of life.

Surrender to the essence in your body.

Feel yourself at home on earth.

Feel the billions of cells in your body at home
on earth.

As you exhale, let go of worries and fear.

You   are   alive   and   you   feel
good . . .   .

THE WORLD OF THE SELF

We are of the earth and mind and spirit compounded.

The Creation Of Health

Our lives are the world. They reflect the vibrations of our entire being. With each gesture, each aware word and thoughtful deed, we express ourselves and create health. We are artists and our life — our creation. We work, weave and sculpt with our daily lives. And even though our world has expanded so that we know its happenings to its most distant corners, the substance of our creation is here — in our lives.

While I write this evening, with the wind rustling in the leaves as the moon wanes, I am flooded with impressions of how circumstances in the mandala of my life have molded me. Yet I can see that while all the configurations of my life have changed — my body, home, family, friends, my ideas — there is at the core of that mandala a creative center that is ever my comforter, my surety, my basis.

I have just arrived home. Part of my homecoming dance is to look toward the Pacific coast around Bodega that I so love. I have danced through the cities and wandered through the deserts only to find the depths of my soul and the altar of my heart.

I left home at fourteen because I had no home within me. It was 1963, and I felt an overwhelming urge to get out from under a way of life threatening my survival. I was depleted by drugs, bored with school, saddened at home; and I had an irrepressible urge to find something better. I stopped using all drugs, including sugar and tobacco. I wandered. I began to open to the healing powers of nature. I began to hear the call of healing. I felt a renewal in my soul.

I helped establish communities where people could be themselves. I thought then that leaving the city was very important for survival. I urged, I preached, that people leave the city, unaware that it was not the city that was the villain but a state of consciousness. (Somewhat later I watched people create the same "city problems" for themselves in the country. It was just nicer — and available to those with money or more options.) It slowly dawned on me that the conflict of our times was one that had to be attended to through processes that did not lend themselves to any simplistic notions, however noble and idealistic.

I began studying systems of medicine. I became deeply involved in various naturopathic orientations. I began a thorough study of vital biological processes, of purification and dietary systems. I studied the use of herbs, water, light.

But my true learning began when I discovered that while biological purification and subsequent grounding in holistic nutrition could initiate the onset of health, real health would only flow from a purity of the heart.

Now, after fifteen years of involvement in natural healing, my work is a direct result of what I have come to realize is its most important component — inspiration. While I often begin with a focus on nutrition, my principal focus is on the spirit in the body. I work with the body as a vehicle for the spirit to express itself in daily life. I attune to the entire being: inspiration is literally a breathing in. I sense the cells spinning. I take guidance from the creative spirit.

Daily inspiration, the daily power to create, can come from the simple basics of our life. Sunrise inspires me. Its light draws me out of bed and I go to a nearby hill where an old windmill still works. I wash with cold water.

The crows that fly over my home morning and evening inspire me. Their flapping wings lift me too. My next-door neighbor inspires me. She loves her child. Sensing their secret bond inspires me. My friends inspire me. The way they work and love and care inspires me.

The vagabond on the highway with a gunny sack of rags over his shoulder — grey beard flapping in the wind — inspires me. The courage of Blacks to remain human even in San Quentin prison inspires me.

Music inspires me. The heartbeat of the tamboura, the drums of the American Indians, the praises to Jah of the Rastafarians, the droning prayers of my grandfather, the blues of Leadbelly, the cooing of children everywhere inspire me.

This daily inspiration empowers us to create our health, for it is *our* creation, *our* unique expression of ourselves. It is the urge of creation that empowers us. Its source? — the life spirit within every cell and every atom of our body. We are all plugged into the one life current running through the earth, vitalizing the food and water, giving us our flesh and form that embody the spirit.

And we contact this power of creation by creating! Since it is within us, we have only to acknowledge its presence for it to manifest. It is with this power that we create health in our lives. And we require no course of self-improvement to discover it. We already have it.

How fascinating and miraculous are the diverse ways in which human beings utilize their power! How life can nourish — and deplete! How some people work with grace and dignity no matter what their task or lot — while others grumble every step they take. While some give wholeheartedly, others are miserly. While some seek companions, others lie alone in dark rooms. While some eat for hunger, others hunger to eat.

Yet every human expression manifests the power of creation, no matter how distorted it must be to surface under onerous conditions. Even the loner is making a statement, even the cynic is crying out. And it is this power that gives us the strength to endure, for it can never be taken away from us. It will resist — and often transcend — the "demands" of fate, the intersections of "our stars," and the lines on our hand. It is affected, but is is often magnificently unconcerned, by what we eat for breakfast, our birth or family, or the ghetto or garden we grow up in.

This power of creation is a faith in life, faith in its beauty and sanctity, and with it we create health in our lives. Daily life is the twenty-four-hour cycle that encompasses the bio-rhythms which our glands, organs, and cells dance to. It is the womb-sleep-darkness-birth-sunrise-activity world. It is a cycle that includes fasting and eating, procreation and solitude, love and work.

It is our work to make well-being daily — by serving creation through loving gently and strongly. We serve creation with every gesture of kindness. We serve creation by protecting Mother Earth, for her waters are our blood, her air our spirit.

Protecting the mother and child serves creation. Planting seeds; tromping through the rice fields; harvesting the corn (their tassels singing in the wind); serving and eating the seeds from which life sprouts; providing the grain for the bread, the tortilla, the matzo, the pasta; making the food for joyous sharing — surely these serve creation.

And we are serving creation when we help mothers secure the space to birth their children in an atmosphere of love and sensitivity; when we feed our children by the principles of holistic nutrition; when we reclaim our bodies from the stereotypes that deaden us; and when we turn away from drugs and weapons to a responsibility for what we produce and what we consume.

And are we not serving creation when we feel the yearning and struggle in the flesh, blood, and hearts of those in need? So is it serving creation to work for liberation — so that the gift of life will not be hoarded, and ghettos, reservations, and concentration camps torn down. Surely it is serving creation to end oppression.

Surely it is serving creation to pierce the shadows of our mind, to feel the sun's rays beaming for all sojourners on our planet, to be attuned with nature, to enjoy the gift of life, to become aware that all is truly one . . .so that we can delight in the simple things, the children, the flowers, our inner music, our needed work.

Again: daily life is truly the form, as our bodies are the vehicle, for the expression of our creativity. The *content* of a *creative* daily life then becomes our response to those gestating forces and movements in our culture seeking to serve creation; and when we do respond, when we do participate in the surge of new energies, we then begin to establish a wholistic consciousness in all areas of our life.

If our daily lives are not the vehicle for our creation, for our participation in the oneness, then we will rely on cures that could magically end war and hunger, clear up pollution, heal the cancers, and calm the distressed. And we will yearn and hope as more and more of the goodness of this earth spoils before our eyes.

But that is not the direction ever-larger numbers of aware people are headed. They have already seen the future (in part) for themselves; and they know it can work for all. Their ally in daily life — as in health-creation — is contact with their Essential Being, with their inner self.

In fact there is no distinction between health-making and daily creation. Health becomes an expression of our being and is therefore unique. It is not in essence a signature of the physical body: it is a *quality* of being, a quality that lives as creation lives with our body.

Health becomes grace; and being, "dying by loving." (Meher Baba.)

Bio-Elemental Healing

A Preface and a Prayer

For each element I sing praise . . .

O air we need you to make
the fire burn
O water we need you to make
the moon turn
O light we need you to make
the planets sing
O earth we need you to make
the spirit ring . . .

Writing about nature is so far from experiencing nature! And yet thoughts — as energy forms, as mental forces — *are* capable of reminding us of our own nature.

Our nature constantly experiences itself. Our minds, often totally preoccupied with other matters, make us unaware that we live and breathe without needing to think to remember to live and breathe. We just do. Thank God! Breathing is our nature. It is our nature to take air into our lungs that has been vitalized by plants. Since our nature is able to do these innate functions without thought, they occur naturally and constantly. This is our basic nature.

But now we must "think air" in order to survive. We must think about how we can save the air so that our grandchildren will be able to breathe. In times past people *had* to breathe because they had to walk. And they had to eat whole food because the processing plants were not in operation. But now it is necessary for survival to learn how to breathe and eat.

In medicine, also, it is necessary to attune to basic functions such as eating and breathing. So it is that bio-elemental healing is actualized by attuning to the basic protoplasmic functions which the four elements (earth, water, air, fire) initiate inside our organism when they are utilized with honor. Yet the four elements mean nothing if they are not realized by the fifth element, the spiritual power of the One. From the One comes the four elements and from the four elements comes our body and the natural optimism of Life.

It is with the fifth element that human beings can cherish and honor nature. Without the experience of the fifth element human beings ail. Now medical treatment relies on chemical drugs, surgery, and psycho-manipulation to heal this ailing. But it cannot be done. It is impossible because it denies the essential nature of our being.

When I ail, I end up going to the Essential Oneness, which is everywhere, in every living thing.

As soon as I REMEMBER and get out of my ailing enough to REMEMBER, I go there. I go to that deep place inside myself where peace is. I go to the Sun and water. I bow my head to the peasant feet of our earth mother. All life is sparked by the essential oneness.

The essence lives in the water and sun in the green plants, and its roots in the fruit and vegetables of this bountiful earth. And when I ail, I go to the Essence to receive the healing that lives there. The result is that the essence in matter and the essence in my being touch — and a circle forms!

That circle girding me, the world, and the Essential Oneness is a healing circle. Do you *feel* what I mean? Healing is being in this circle and allowing creation to be.

Exploration and Theory

First a plea, a reaching out to you, dear reader, for patience with our attempts to soar high enough over our beautiful, troubled earth to encompass this wordless subject we call bio-elemental healing so that we might finally land on the earth again with enough under-standing and aspiration to begin the actual ancient practice of this healing art.

Why the attempt to soar? Because bio-elemental healing is so basic in its celebration of our biological foundations that it demands an intuitive perspective to be comprehended. It demands a biologi-cal mysticism to apprehend the body as a medium through which we receive and translate all our nurturing and our healing. With such heightened awareness healing becomes a communion with God's speech to humanity: the protoplasmic wisdom coded into our cells.

It is very difficult to turn toward new healing ways. It is hard to receive nature where buildings cast eternal shadows, but it is within our power to initiate the healing response no matter where we are.

We had better do it.

Our survival depends on it. By the year 2000, two out of four people will contract cancer, and one-sixth of all animal species will be extinct if their present rate of destruction continues. Wouldn't it be strange if mysticism became a survival necessity! Perhaps we need a new definition of "mysticism". Is something mystical if it happens, if it is real, if at least parts of it are palpable and evident, and if it is predictable — even though it cannot be linguistically explained?

But actually people are doing it, they are turning toward nature and away from our tremendously complex medical system that "scientifically" purveys chemicalized medicine, needless surgery, and psycho-manipulation. The special horror is the pain and viola-tion visited upon patients with degenerative diseases — cancer, heart disease, arthritis, etc.

The domain of bio-elemental healing *is* nature! It utilizes the primal healing forces in the biological states of matter (earth, water, air, sun) and their corresponding psychological aspects by contacting the appropriate element to release controlling thought patterns. It is a holistic system that focuses *through* the body-mind to the unified spiritual energy at the source of all creation.

Actually, the energy in the states of matter has correlating functions within human beings so that it can be utilized to facilitate their natural healing capabilities. (All healing — whether from pill or knife, or the four elements must derive ultimately from the pristine power of nature.)

Indeed all the different forms of nature and all the various changes that the states of matter undergo (including those inside our body) are visible surfaces of this unified energy. The visualization of brain, organs, and glands and the resurgence of our basic optimistic nature can only be accomplished with the intervention of this healing force.

Contact with the wisdom of this primal energy that programs the cells to live, metabolize and regenerate has ever been a vitalizing, stabilizing, and healing force for human beings. It has ever been a natural way to experience the unified power of creation. Many of the activities of daily life formerly provided this elemental contact and its associated "primary process" thinking that often accompanies revery.

But now we do not have enough contact with our natural selves. Increasingly, our lives are spent either in our heads (thinking, scheming, worrying, coping) or else pursuing "entertaining" ways of shaking loose (drugs, disco, guru-hopping). Yet human beings cannot live separate from nature without incurring disease.

That is why bio-elemental healing is also the *medical* expression of the transformation many are now experienceing in their entire life orientation. This approach in healing is an important antidote to experiences of birth trauma, emotional confusion, lifelong ingestion of chemicalized foods, and psychic tension. It is appropriate medicine for our fragmented times since it utilizes the life force and so meets our holistic needs. It is a true application of ecological consciousness.

The transformation from the medical establishment's allopathic consciousness, geared to drugs and surgery, to healing practices focused on the biochemical requirements of the cellular structure (naturopathic nutrition) and the need to dispense with crippling behavior patterns is happening at an amazing rate. This profoundly changed perspective sees human beings as essentially peaceful, loving, sharing, and creative if they are provided with the opportunity to experience their natural selves, to truly immerse in the "power world" of nature, and to participate in redeeming social rituals.

Bio-elemental healing is grounded in the understanding that only nature heals. And we are nature. Oneness is. And so we turn toward healing ways that honor our essential integrity. We turn toward new healing ways with the understanding that ways of creating well-being are not the spin-offs of sophisticated reasoning. They are not the property of any school of thought. Nor are they special to certain people. They are common sense held in common to create (literally!) more common sense.

Why do people go down to the ocean? Why is there a lust to splash in water? (that only children are "foolish" enough to satisfy). Why do people sail?

Why do people garden, mow the lawn, pot flowers? Once again: why do children make mud pies? Why does the earth seem rich and mysterious?

Why do the rich go off to Switzerland or the Bavarian Alps? Why does the first snowfall send children into a frenzy of delight?

Why do people need to get some air, to take a walk, to somehow breathe in the universe if they're angry or sad or frustrated — or rapturously in love?

Why do people stare at a fire for hours? Why will they travel for hours to get to a beach — for a short interval of sun? What is the magic in flame?

Who knows exactly? No one does, of course. But really everyone knows what we're talking about. If you are at all confused by the abstractness of our words, this is fundamentally all we really mean by bio-elemental healing.

Please hold on to these examples of natural healing as we go on to describe theory and ways of relating to the four elements in order to commune with the pristine energy of matter.

The Earth

Obeisance to the Mother

Hsin t'u wu Chi. The word in Chinese for ecology translates:
"body earth not two"

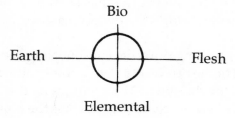

I will honor the earth and remember it is the source of all my material comforts. I will honor the earth by delighting in her bounty, by walking barefoot on the dewy morning grass, by taking refuge in her green coolness. I will honor the earth by protecting her from the ravages of the greedy and foolish.

The physical earth is our body. Actually. Literally. Dynamically. We are creatures of *this* very particular and blessed sphere. All our glands and organs and rhythms are connected to the cycles of this earth plane. Without the bounty of the earth I would not have the privilege to communicate in this way. The paper, the energy used in publishing are derived from the earth. I pray that all these words have an effect in saving our earth.

To align with the earth plane, one honors the nutritional process as a fundamental way of attunement. It is not "just a personal thing" to take care of one's own body. Honoring the nutritional process is honoring the energy that has been provided us to thrive on; and only by honoring this energy can we begin to live in harmony.

Furthermore, healing ourselves and healing the earth are one and the same. The health of the soil is the health of the people. People that care for the soil — by giving it its due — safeguard their own vitality. When chemicals despoil the soil, the people's health degenerates. It hurts the earth to produce foods at its expense. Food grown by agribusiness to be processed, refined, and chemicalized exploits both the people and the earth. Healing can only be accomplished through a natural and mutual exchange with nature.

In the Upanishads, one of the oldest cherished writings of humanity, it is said, "First know food, from food all things are born, by food they live, toward food they move, into food they return."

Ways of Attunement

1.   Earth meditation: O, dear mother, please guide me so that my life may be in harmony with your needs. As I walk, make me conscious of those who toil in the fields and factories so that I might eat. As I walk, inspire me with your incredible endurance so that I may help you in your work of sustaining humanity.
2.   A direct way of exchanging energy with the earth is to apply clay to the body. It draws out the poisons!
3.   Another way is to place the naked body in contact with the earth — whether at the beach or on grass or ground. We allow ourselves thus to be magnetized by the earth — and so stabilized!

Water

Obeisance to the Flow

We begin our life in the amniotic waters of the womb, whose composition is much like the ocean.

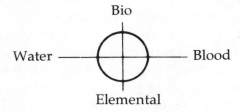

Water ——— Blood

Bio

Elemental

Cellular Meditation: I will be with the river of my life, flowing through birth and death, flowing through flesh and blood, flowing through time and infinity, flowing through form and spirit.

mind can be seen. She holds teary sadness and angry torrents. She is the easy flow of the stream moving along on the way to the ocean. She is direct, unstoppable. She is the pool, hanging back in reflection.

Water fills the vessels of plants and is made alive. Water is the blood of the earth. Water becomes red blood and green chlorophyll. Water is alive. To drink pure water is soothing for the body.

Ways of Attunement

1.   Water Meditation: Feel the nature of water, the flowingness, and find that place in yourself, that place that flows no matter what your current crisis; that place that flows gently and naturally. Now take yourself to some water (actual or imaginary). Hear it, whispering. Now bathe youself, and as you do, feel your concerns and troubles being washed away. Let the water soothe and cleanse you. Let the water surround you, lighten you, hold you. Let the water teach you. Let the water heal you.

2.   Healing with water is called hydrotherapy. Unfortunately, hot water is considered most therapeutic in our culture; and yet, although relaxing, it is generally weakening to the organism. It is much overused. Cool water is stimulating, draws blood to the surface, and strengthens the organism. Cold water can improve the absorptive power of the gastric and intestinal mucous membranes, thereby aiding the nutritional process. It has a two-fold effect: It slows the circulation where it is applied; but then when the application stops, increased function occurs. (Hot water, on the other hand, dilates arteries, veins, and lymph channels.)

   a. Take a soothing bath in your home: just add apple cider vinegar or sea salt — thus restoring the proper alkaline-acid balance for the skin. Another u   ful addition is Glauber's Salts.

   b. A most beneficial treatment is alternating hot and cold water.

   c. Warm water deeply massaged into the body is very healing.

   d. Listen to water! It makes a soothing music.

Air

Obeisance to the Vital Spaciousness

In Hebrew the words for breath (*nephesh* and *ruakh*) mean the essence of life.

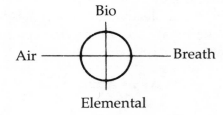

> I will give myself the spaciousness in which to fulfill my creativity and will alllow others to be creative in their lives. I will delight each day in the holy essence of air and consciously connect my breaths like pearls on a necklace.

Air is our most essential food.Without it life expires.And yet how we have betrayed our need for this vital substance. We have closed ourselves off from the power of air. In our homes, cities, schools, and workplace there is no fresh air. Is it any wonder that few of us breathe deeply anymore? Who wants a mouthful of cigarette smoke or gasoline exhaust? Who wants their lungs full of over-heated or chilled air? Where we live affects how we breathe, and how we breathe affects where we live. As we cherish the angel of life in the air, we will purify the air — and cherish ourselves!

Being aware of our breathing provides a means of connecting our autonomic and parasympathetic nervous systems; it puts us in charge of our lives. By attuning to our breath we become sensitive to the world like a mother who knows the breathing of her own child. What is our breath saying? Is it shallow and irregular? Is it quick and halting? Is it steady and flowing? By attuning to ourselves through the breath we are brought into contact with the source of healing.

Ways of Attunement

1. Air Meditation: Go out into the morning air to visit growing plants. As you breathe, feel yourself filling with vitality. Feel this vitalness, this life-force energy, spread throughout your entire being, into your flesh and blood, all the way into your cells. Picture your cells spinning, and as they spin hear them singing and rejoicing for life.

2. Harmonic breath — walking can be very centering if we coordinate our movement with the breath. Just take four steps on the inhale and four steps on the exhale. Simple.

3. The exhale is more important than the inhale. If we exhale completely, new air will come in naturally. Only by letting go of the past can we experience the present.

4. Sleeping in well ventilated rooms (or outside when the weather permits) affords the greatest opportunity for a truly rejuvenating rest.

5. Here's a breath relaxer: inhale six counts, then exhale six. It will put you to sleep too!

6. Cells that have ample oxygen do not develop cancer.

The Sun

Obeisance to the Light

. . . and there was light

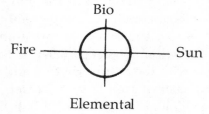

I will allow myself to feel and express the love in my heart and will receive and appreciate the love vibrations of others.

— from Okute or Shooter, speaking of his holy beliefs —

"All living creatures and all plants derive their life from the sun. If it were not for the sun, there would be darkness and nothing could grow — the earth would be without life. Yet the sun must have the help of the earth."

The sun is the heart of our universe. The sun is the mother of our earth. The sun is our daily ally as we journey toward health.

Our relationship with the light of the sun greatly affects our ability to sleep just as our ability to sleep greatly affects our ability to waken. Sleep is like the exhale in breathing: to awaken, to breathe in new life, we must sleep. Sleep is the time when our organism connects with the cosmic rhythm and is renewed. If we respond to the rhythm of sunrise and sunset, we can also synchronize with our biological clock which still ticks in primordial harmony with the light and darkness.

The sun's vibrations — colors — constantly enliven us. Goethe called them "the suffering of light". Since they are different wavelengths, they have subtly different — though profound — effects. We are uplifted by the blues of the sky and water, balanced and soothed by the green of leaves and grass, and given hope and inspiration by the yellow, orange, and purple of flowers.

While working on patients' bodies in my healing practice, I will often have them visualize colors as they breathe. (I have learned to sense the appropriate colors for soothing or invigorating. I can then ask that they inhale a specific color and exhale another.)

One of the most essential solar therapeutics is sun-bathing. After all, the skin is the largest organ in the body, functioning as protector of our internal organs, and as an avenue for elimination and absorption. The proper stimulation of the skin with massage, hydrotherapy, and sun-bathing strengthens the internal organs, especially the kidneys and lungs. The best time for sunbathing is in the morning or afternoon, when the sun's rays are most assimilable.

Ways of Attunement

1.   Meditation on the Sun: Let us go into the morning sun, grateful for the warmth and light and its benediction of hope. Let us stand in awe of the consistent power of the sun. Let us go into the morning sun to align our hearts with the heart of our universe.

2.   We need natural full-spectrum light on our bodies and eyes. This has recently been substantiated by the work of Dr. John Ott. He has found a layer of cells in the retina that absorb light and stimulate the pineal and pituitary glands. The light must be natural. Light that comes through windows, glasses, or excessive air pollutants does not nourish in this way; in fact, it causes mal-illumination.

3.   There is a sun inside our body: our heart. When our awareness involves the heart (in compassion) it is the perfect purifier. So it is that when we are compassionate of our imperfections we can lessen their control.

     Imagine utilizing the purifying effect of fire in this exercise: Take your worries, fears, doubts, and confusions and wrap them in a bundle. Now take this bundle to a fire and throw it in. Watch it burn! That is the fate of everything not of our essence. Dust to dust.

5.   Our attunement to the sun and our ability to utilize its power will determine our survival as a species. If we are to survive the sun will become our main source of energy.

6.   Appreciating the sun is one of the basic ways of appreciating our essential being.

The Art Of Active Dreaming

I have been living a dream for the last few months. Yet I feel closer to reality than I have ever been, for the purpose of dreaming is to help us be real. Dreams are mirrors of our lives, they are nourished in our reality; their purpose is not to waylay us or delude us or scare us. Their purpose is to wake us up — *to our reality*. Don't let their language fool you: they "lie" only to tell the truth.

Let me share my dream with you. I am on a pleasant road through the woods. I'm tired, however, so I sit down on the road to rest when suddenly a car looms at my back. It is going slow but it could break my back.

It's an old car, very old, but it is still dangerous. I have a cane in my hand. I am terrified but speechless. Finally I overcome my fear and raise my cane, shouting, "Stop!"

The old car stops. Then I stand up and feel in control and the dream ends . . .

What does it mean? It's better to say: how does it mean? A dream is like a poem. It "means" with metaphor; and metaphor doesn't speak to us in the ordinary language of reality. Metaphor uses *existential* equations to mirror our life so that we can see it — in part — as a spectator, and learn. Metaphor is a likeness without the "like"; it takes a leap and says we *are* something else. It combines idea and feeling in an utterly new view of our reality. Metaphor is the language of poem . . .and dream. When we learn to understand our poetry, we wake up to life.

For example, if a strong man is called a bull and a beautiful child a flower, we know something more about each than strength and beauty. Although "bull" and "flower" are cliches, there is still an important "charged idea" in the information they purvey. "Bull" and "flower" have existential impact.

But what about the metaphor of dreams? If only the information dreams purvey were that accessible! Yet it is available even though most people think it outlandish, weird, and often scary — and therefore dismissible. But we dismiss it at great cost, for our very being speaks in the dream about the essence of our life. And we can re-learn the language of our hidden speech.

What did *my* dream mean? That I am tired of would's (woods! — my dreams pun fiendishly: my road is generally bordered with heavy expectations!) and my habitual ways of using my energy (my old car, that is) will break my back unless I raise cain (cane!)

I *have* been raising cain, I have been calling my critical, nagging inner "computer" sternly to task — and it's been working, I have been living better. I feel freer. I know now *through doing* that it is helpful to be summarily angry at my old patterns. I regularly fantasize my dream helper* obliterating my old car — which I then trade in for a Porsche. I run more smoothly, and I'm in the driver's seat! I have much more energy and more enthusiasm.

Just a "simple dream" perhaps. I have had hundreds such — many far more significant. Yet it is amazing how even it can light up one's life, to its farthest horizon!

Kilton Stewart, who adapted the Senoi dream system for Western use, said it best: "Perhaps the greatest dream which man has created, from the beginning of time up to the present, is the theory that each man's mind can and should be free to think or dream to any distance in any direction."

It's true that Western tradition has encouraged *thought* in any direction. *But to dream, to use* this capacity to revisualize our life so that we can change it in surprisingly creative directions? No, here we have been discouraged. In fact, our tradition has derided the dream so that it is necessary to retrieve its amazing power — and therefore wise to invoke those individuals *in our tradition* who re-discovered its truth and its value, and actually have dreamt to any distance in any direction.

---

*'This concept will be explained later.

Poe's poems and short stories, for example, are often barely this side of the drawn drapes of sleep. And Coleridge barely parted the drapes with his "Kubla Khan," recovering 54 dream-inspired lines (of the 200-300 he had originally envisioned) before he was unfortunately interrupted.

Robert Louis Stevenson not only parted the drapes but converted his dream mind into a plot-producing factory in which his "Brownies" (as he put it) concocted successful stories as he slept — the most renowned being "The Strange Case of Dr. Jekyll and Mr. Hyde."

Kekule realized the benzene ring from a dream, thus revolutionizing modern chemistry. Afterward he recalled that he had had similar dreams previously but had not been aware of their import. (Recurring dreams need not be nightmares!) No wonder he concluded a speech to colleagues with the remark, "Let us learn to dream, gentlemen, and then we may perhaps find the truth."

Why is it then that the use of dreams has been accorded little sanction in modern times until perhaps quite recently? A full answer could take a book! But — very briefly — the rationalistic approach to life ushered in by the Industrial Revolution was largely responsible. It was not then understood that a non-rational (not *irrational*) mode of being, like dreams, could — by virtue of its inner vision — offer a deeply needed inner view of our "other-directed" way of life.

And so the impetus to decipher dreams died, their ways forgotten, their language almost lost. At best they reminded us that we had eaten unwisely or that lechery still lurked underneath our civilized disguise... Until recently.

Until Jung, Perls, and Stewart showed that dreams are reflections of the self in its transit through life and that all persons and objects and conditions in dreams are parts and phases of the self. Stewart* advanced further than Jung and Perls: he has shown Western dreamers that we can control our dreams, that we can shape our dreams so that they will not only explain the voyage of the self through life but re-map the voyage! Thus the dream changes life as life changes the dream in continous interchange.

---

*I am deeply indebted to Stewart and his widow, Clara Stewart Flagg, who has carried on his work indefatiguably, for much of the substance of this chapter.

To make this contribution Stewart had one important advantage over his predecessors: he was an anthropologist and so was not committed to any psychological theory nor, therefore, blinded from appreciating the Senoi dreamers of Malaya who showed him a society with no crime or violence for 300 years and whose "psychotherapy, emotional education, and interpersonal relations are perhaps the most efficient and highly evolved which the human race has yet attained."* And this entire edifice was based on a system of dream education!

Furthermore, its values were in harmony with a Western belief in the primary value of life and a pragmatic and experimental attitude toward improving it so that it could be adapted to a seemingly alien Western culture.

The Senoi simply and affirmatively state (first to the children as soon as they can talk) that all images and thoughts in dreams are good and useful if they are expressed, criticized, and acted on in a social context.

And so it is that at breakfast first priority is given to sharing the previous night's dreams, and particular attention is paid to the children who have not learned how to confront their terror and menace. They are soon taught with the support of father, mother, and the older children to outface and conquer nightmare spirits until they can develop dream allies of their own.

As the children mature, they learn to love and forgive so that they will have helpful dream characters. However, they might have to kill off some non-cooperative dream figures in order to assure a constructive dream life that can promote love and respect in the real world — so that terror dreams usually disappear before puberty, when dream life becomes more realistic, reflective, and constructive.

And since every member of the family group not only evaluates the shared dream symbols but also helps suggest an actual group project to *act* on their meaning, dreaming becomes the main source of creative thinking about technical, artistic, and social problems.

---

*Stewart, Kilton: "How to Educate Your Dreams to Work for You"; pub. 1973 by Clara Stewart Flagg, New York. Page 2.

Actually, the society's outstanding dreamers become so profi-
cient that "stenographers" actually sit by their beds waiting for
poems, songs, dances, ways of fishing and hut-building, and even
new diplomatic approaches to other tribes to be dictated out of
their sleep! In truth, the Senoi have dreamt up their culture.

Naturally, we need to adapt and modify the Senoi way for
modern Western life; nevertheless the essence of the way can
remain because it is based on the proven assumption that dreams
do tell us how to integrate our lives. The problem is — translating
their message and then realizing it in the real world.

The Senoi discovered centuries ago that in the dream, as Perls
put it, "First you look through a window, and suddenly you
recognize that you are just looking in a mirror." For the dream
is — often magically and uncannily — a projection of the
dreamer; therefore the dreamer must repossess and reintegrate the
self's hidden, wayward, and fragmented parts to move on in the
business of living.

Even physiologically the body is almost geared for action in the
dream state. The sympathetic nervous system (which serves activity and survival roles) is close to full functioning: brain waves
closely resemble the waking pattern; adrenalin is firing the system;
there is high sexual arousal, heartbeat and pulse are up — our
energy is running and all systems are close to "Go!"

Isn't it time, then, that we listen to our dreams; that, as the
Talmud says, we consider "a misunderstood dream like an un-
opened letter"?

Isn't it time then that we see the dream as an artistic production
using artistic symbols to speak about the process of living in the
world? We are all artists!

We dream about two hours a night. Isn't it time then that we
wake up to these dreams? Otherwise they can encroach on reality
and poison the essence of both. (A psychotic is someone who
cannot distinguish between the two.)

True, we are all artists; but there is a science to art. However we
can begin simply — yet with total confidence.

Start with a dream notebook (make it ample size and you'll have
"big" dreams!) and a pen or penlight by your bed: you must
convince your dream mind you mean business, or else it won't
cooperate. (The penlight is useful if you have a sleeping partner.)

Treat a dream like a butterfly! When you are aware you have finished a dream, wake up carefully, gently — or else it will fly away. Then review the dream as you lie in various sleeping positions, for often parts of the dream will only be recalled in the position you dreampt them! Handle them with cotton wool and they'll sidle up to you for recall — *for they do want to be acknowledged.* Then write the dream down. (If it's the middle of the night, you will be amazed at how quickly you return to sleep. The reason is that you will have fulfilled an obligation to the oneness, thus facilitating the relaxation process.)

Remember that your dream mind only operates on the basis of credibility. If you want it to help you in a special problem area, then involve yourself with that area for at least two days; then when you go to bed, focus on it up to the last few minutes before falling asleep. Tell your dream mind that you want it to dream to a resolution and that you want it to wake you up so that you can record the dream. It will do so if it believes you!

Once you have recorded the dream narrative, there are three essential questions you need to answer. The first is: how did you feel during the dream? Then: what did you connect with? That is, what did the dream as a whole relate to in your life? (Usually, it refers to the events of the previous day.) The third question is: how would you want to change the dream?

Connections should also be made with any dream symbols that seem puzzling or foreign. Let yourself go. Freely associate. Your unconscious knows the answer — allow your marvelous "computer" to work! (we are referring to pesonal symbols: "universal" and cultural symbols we shall be discussing later, although your computer will likely know them too.)

For example, I dreamt the night before writing this that I was driving a car on a wide boulevard and would have to turn left on Time Avenue to attend a meeting of the Hardware Workers Union, which was contemplating a strike.

I will only deal with my connections with the world "left." There were two possibilities *for me.* The first that came to mind (and that is the one we should usually go with) is that of relaxation, intuition, of the "feminine" side of my nature — which I often neglect when I am wearing myself hard (hardware!).

The other association is the political left. But perhaps the two meanings fused! for the Union seems to be in radical mood and wants to strike against the oppression of my "Rightist" tendencies (my rigid, "hard-wearing," driving, and judging). Well what's wrong with a coalition of both lefts?

Another dimension of recording a dream is translating it into artistic media, such as poetry, narrative, painting, sculpture, etc. But "translating" is misleading, for the dream in essence *is* an artistic production that uses narrative, scenic atmosphere, and animate and inanimate symbols to shed light on and give direction to the life of the dreamer.

So you will have to answer two questions in your "translation": Will you want to change the symbolism enough so that it can be grasped by others in order to make a "public" dream? Or is the translation mainly for your benefit? — so that you can preserve the dream in a form that can help recall its personal significance.

To dream to any distance requires that we be responsible to any distance for our dreams. As a child, for example, Stevenson was paralyzed by nightmares and struggled to stay awake so that he would not have to face them. He would often find himself awake "clinging to the curtain rod with his knees to his chin."

Even as medical student, they scourged him until he consulted a doctor who enabled him to see that he could take charge of his dreams since *he* dreamt them. After that they were no longer hostile external agents but his own productions: he had finally defused them.

But he hadn't harnessed them as yet, and so occasionally they could still be quite troubling. He then began putting himself to sleep with tales of his own making — elaborating on them, changing them, then dropping them for new creations, all purely for his own pleasure and relaxation.

Then something curious and significant happened after he decided to become a professional storyteller. You will recall we said that the dream mind does not recognize credibility gaps; however it was obviously credible to it that he meant business when he began searching for plots in his professional endeavors — for he had been "plotting" with its help for a long time. So his "Brownies" got busy. He describes (in the third person) their activity:

..."the little people begin to bestir themselves in the same quest, and labour all night long, and all night long set before him truncheons of tales upon their lighted theatre. No fear of his being frightened now."...

We can learn from Stevenson. Isn't our dream mind already a storyteller par excellence? But unfortunately sometimes we don't appreciate how the stories turn out. They can be scary, threatening, malicious, destructive, paralyzing. A "bad" dream can wipe us out for a day or two, even scar our memory for life, seeping through the psyche to our very marrow. But on the other hand a "good" dream will fuel us with powerful energy that will accomplish difficult projects with ease and make us buoyant and hopeful: a boon for our being.

This is where we need to start in our dream work, for as of now we must become convinced that "bad" and "good" are irrelevant designations and that all dreams are essentially good though they might have uncomfortable feelings to report. If they do have, we need to know it so that we can use our energies more profitably; but we need not *identify* with those feelings. A nightmare, as Perls put it, simply shows us how we are frustrating ourselves; and we can correct that and control it once we know we're doing it.

There are three ascending levels of dream control: We can re-fantasize the dream. We can re-dream it. Or, ultimately, we can "preside" over our dreams *as they happen*, to bring about immediate creative results.

However, the starting point for all three levels is the same utterly proven belief that we can take charge of our psychic life. Actually re-fantasizing and re-dreaming are closely related processes.

In fact, you will discover that when you re-fantasize you will often "go over" into a dreamlike state. In any case the distinction between fantasy and dream is not crucial since they are sister processes; indeed, exceedingly valuable dream work can be accomplished through fantasy.

Both require that you re-plot the dream and re-enact it in fantasy or dream *to your satisfaction*. What would it be like if your negative dream symbols were converted to positives — perhaps even to allies, so that they would help *you* in a creative mission? After all you *are* their parent!

Ideally, you would re-fantasize or re-dream after waking from an unsatisfying dream. There are two reasons for striking then: the dream is fresh and you are probably in a relaxed state, even though perturbed. However, if you are *highly* anxious or there has been a long interval between the original dream and your "re-play" a relaxation exercise would be advisable.

In that case, do some deep breathing followed by meditation— that is, watch the screen of your mind with attentive objectivity as the flotsam and jetsam in your awareness flow on, and away. Take your time. LET IT GO . . . Give yourself permission to relax.

Then, when you are in tune, fantasize or re-dream yourself into that original dream space so that you can now do away with the animate *and inanimate* negatives in the dream — and we mean "do away with" literally. Nothing is more creative in dream work than love and murder! Bring your operatic self to stage center and let it happen . . .

But before you murder, you must confront the negative — no matter how scary the prospect — for you can make surprising conversions. In any case, you will never die in a dream: you might be "killed," but you will never die. Encounter it, have a dialogue with it, outface it. In nine times out of ten the lion will become a pussy cat; the malevolent beast, a lamb; the demon, a shy friend! Try it — it works. Remember: you are the master of your dream world. But if the villain will not recant, wipe (him, her, it) out totally!

Which reminds me of a dream I had just as I was finishing the book — this particular dream work being my last writing. (I should point out I was very tired: it was a hard — but good — pull.)....

I am in my car with my wife, Betty, in the rear seat. I am extremely tired. I have been driving a long distance. Now I am coming on the main street of a city, waiting to make a left turn. I inch forward, but then a huge truck lumbers by, forcing me to back up.

I then inch forward again, and again another massive truck roars by, compelling me to go back slightly. Now I get on the main street, but I realize I'm dead tired and begin pushing the car forward with my feet — all the time being highly indignant at my wife for not offering assistance.

Finally my fatigue and frustration freeze my will to move, and I decide to stop, as the dream ends.

Fortunately, I had the time to re-dream! But first let's look at the key symbols I had to use or convert in order to make the dream a productive one. To begin with, my car is my energy system, and *that's* rather low; in fact it needs to be pushed to move at all.

My wife Betty? She, of course, symbolizes a part of me since all symbols in the dream represent parts and aspects of the dreamer. I think of her as dynamic, spontaneous and joyful. but she's at my rear and unused, though a part of me...

So in my first re-dream I had *her* drive — whereupon she quickly drove out to the country to an idyllic grassy meadow where we made love, bringing into the world a lovely child, Connie (from Constance!), whom I quickly matured to a young woman for a future dream helper.

I also had a dialogue with Betty in the re-dream when she poined out how impossible I am when I play martyr! She described my sighs and groans punishingly well! I then pointed out that I didn't trust her to drive because she's so sure of herself and makes it so easy. (I do tend to make life a struggle.) But I realized that when I allowed her to drive, she drove for *me.*

Therefore I decided to drive my own car, with her in the front seat supporting *me.* After all, I became aware, I needed to focus my energy — I needed to do my own driving.

So, on a second re-dream, off we went again. As I held her hand, she sitting happily next to me, something beautiful occurred. She merged with me, we coalesced, so that now we were together. (Incidentally, we were now in a new Porsche.) I felt strengthened and happy. I also decided I *could* take time off to rest.

Obviously, there are many elements in the dream I have not gone into — like those lumbering trucks, for example. But the main point is: confront the dream, it is your dream; so make it *truly* yours.

So first, confront your negatives. Even if they obdurately hold on to their hostility, you must dialogue with them, experience them; for they might have something important to tell you. Then, if necessary, kill them off. But don't leave the corpses lying around to clutter your dream world — incinerate them and then fertilize a beautiful plant or useful crop. Make your dreams productive projects.

If it is at all possible, alter a negative part so that it *can* be made love to. Love is a superior force in the dream world too. Make love to all positives of whatever sex — or whatever relationship to you. Remember that *all symbols in a dream are parts of you* and that therefore you will not be defying a moral code in the real world if you make love to your mother or father or brother or friend. Not only make love: if at all possible, love through orgasm to birth a new ally who can work for you in your dream world. Lovers of your own sex can give birth too!

Then age your child in a matter of seconds to maturity so that it can work for you. Allies are marvelously useful, especially for all the "dirty work" that needs to be done. It is especially potent to parent positives with traits that you don't sufficiently demonstrate in the real world. For example, I have an ally who is ruthlessly decisive. He can assassinate and demolish my most cherished hangups with the swish of the cleaver, the spurt of a flame thrower, or the silence of a ray gun! I also have a female ally who offers surcease and support in stress. And they are both aspects of me! I, of course, have many other figures who can prevail when I need them. Most I have named and can recall them to duty readily . . .

There are also inanimate negatives that need to be dealt with. We are everything in the dream: flowers, sky, grass, ocean, rocks, mountains, deserts, filing cases, bureaus, desks and refrigerators, rooms, apartment houses. Everything that is hard and rigid, that compartmentalizes and encloses, or that is lifeless and sterile must go.

Ask yourself: "What in my life is rocklike and stubborn? How can I work through these rigidities?" Then pulverize the rocks into fruitful soil and convert the mountains to tillable land — in fantasy or dream. Filing cases, refrigerators, apartment houses, etc., must be annihilated also. But first find out what parts of your psyche you are filing away, or putting into cold storage, or compartmentalizing!

Bowel movements in a dream are liberating. They indicate a letting-go of hangups, anger, resentment. Think of the hangups and resentments you want to get rid of and then fantasize and/or dream psychological bowel movements that will fertilize the soil with your hangups! (You can cure yourself of constipation, ulcers, and hemorrhoids with just such preventive care.)

The Senoi system is activist, creative, and constructive. Allow no games or carnivals in the dream world. (They are, of course, most necessary in the real world.) If you are flying, fly *somewhere* and come back with a discovery, with a new feeling for the universe, with an enriched sense of beauty.

If you are falling, fall and land before you wake up! You will be all right. It's just a dream and you are in charge. Imagine yourself on a space mission: bring back a sample of the terrain, a report of the vegetation and animal life or of the people you meet; record the colors, the sounds, the activities you experience.

It is essential to confront and conquer danger. Once again: *You* cannot die, though an aspect or part of you may be "killed." In fact, in dreams death is auspicious, for it is the underside of the eternal cycle of destruction and renewal. You can then immediately be reborn as a more vital being. Indeed, doctors, nurses, hospitals — symbols of human malfunction and disease — are superfluous in the dream world. They are energy drains. Kill off the sick, destroy the faulty so that renewed parts of yourself in the dream world can revitalize your self and your life in the real world.

You must also realize that you have — or will soon have — allies in the dream world whom you can call on to zap any enemy — no matter how formidable or vicious. After all, your cohorts will have ray guns, neutron bombs, disintegrators, flame throwers, machine guns, steamrollers, shredders, and slingshots in their armory. What "dire" enemy could withstand such abuse!

But don't stop. After your "foe" has been conquered and subdued, require tribute — demand a gift. (You *ask* a dream lover for a gift after orgasm; but from a fear-producing symbol you *demand* one.) A positive resolution to the dream is your first concern. A gift, a guide, a poem, a plan — all are outcomes that indicate you are master of the people and forces in your dream and therefore have — or can insure — the approval of all parts of yourself. For after all, the goal is still oneness: a reintegrated self that can stand tall and strong in the dream world — and therefore ultimately in the real world.

As we have said, the first two levels of dream control are, first, fantasy and then the re-dream (though, as we pointed out, both are often parts of a "seamless" process). Even the master key to dream control — lucid dreaming — cannot be set apart from the other two levels; for you will discover that as you practice the latter your lucidity will emerge.

What is lucidity? It is simply an ongoing awareness that you're dreaming *while you're dreaming*. Actually, all dreamers experience an inkling of this state when we drop over the edge into dream upon first falling asleep: we "know" momentarily where we're going. Likewise, during a fantastic and/or scary dream we will wake up sufficiently to reassure ourselves that it is a dream, and thus will experience — if not pure lucidity — at least the feeling of both states.

What happens then, in most cases, is that we either wake up totally or simply fall asleep and so shut off entry to dream control — and we are so close at this point. since lucidity is a peculiar product of both the conscious and unconscious states. If you know you're dreaming, there is no longer any terror since you have one foot in reality, as it were, while you're exploring your dream world.

However, these inklings to lucidity — which we generally call pre-lucid states — can help us achieve full lucidity. For example, several times a day you can tell yourself that "dreams are only dreams" until eventually you will know it and remember it during a dream. Another good statement is: "This is a dream and I can wake up to it." You can and you will.

We also spoke about that transitional point of pre-lucidity where one drops off into dream. We need then to test reality while at the same time remaining in the dream stage. We need to say (especially at this point also): "This is a dream and I can wake up to it."(That is, we can be lucid, we can be aware, while dreaming.)

We need to extend those moments of lucidity that we all share. For example, we have all experienced telling ourselves that "it was just a dream" as we woke up from a fantastic, frustrating, or scary experience. Now we can tell ourselves this while dreaming. Take control, take charge, direct and stage-manage your dream in the "theatre," right on stage. It's only a dream. You can stay asleep and wake up to it.

It has become banal to compare the world to a stage and ourselves to actors. What is it then to compare a dream to a play? Isn't it? It is not real. Its sole purpose is to make our lives real — to extract all that we can from our lives based on all that we are. The dream aims to reveal ourselves in action by showing us how we live through dream symbolism.

When we achieve lucidity, when you know you're dreaming, then your dreams will become more realistic. That is a turning point. No longer will your dream mind have to startle you or scare you or torture you to get you to pay attention to your life, for it will know that you *are* — and so have become a mature dreamer.

The main caution is — don't become too emotionally involved or else this realistic phase will end. Remember: you are in charge and it's only a dream.

Before you arrive at the realistic symbolism of lucid dreaming, however, you will be facing the problem of interpreting your symbols. Actually, you will discover it is not a disabling problem since you will know what most symbols mean in context with the dream as a whole, especially in relation to the feelings that it generates and the people and things the feelings connect with.

If you have any doubts, have a dialogue with the symbol (animate or inanimate) and ask "it" to reveal itself. It is often helpful to "be" the person or thing you confront. Act out your own symbols — you will know what to say in their behalf, for they are truly parts of you that you have not integrated fully in your life and which, therefore, *want to speak in your behalf.*

Yet some symbols do have well-nigh universal application — although most are culturally and/or personally derived — so that it is helpful to recognize the significance of a symbol when you meet it. For this reason the following brief list is appended with one essential caution: if the significance and disposition suggested don't fit or seem relevant, use your own. You are the prime authority! The idea is to work with *your* symbols and to change them if necessary in fantasy or dream.

SYMBOL	SIGNIFICANCE AND/OR DISPOSITION
animals	Obviously this is a huge subject. You'll be able to tell what they mean by confronting them, dialoguing with them. Ants, spiders, dogs, snakes, fish, rats are sex or energy symbols. Chop them up and make a stew out of them — then a totem feast! Seriously, this will be energizing!
authorities	Mother symbols. She was your first absolute monarch, your first authority, wasn't she? How is she still judging, policing, presiding over you? Get rid of her. Remember that by getting rid of her (that is, *your* negative image of her) you will be better able to get along with your real mother.
automobiles	These are your energy systems — highly significant. What model is it? what condition? what color? Is it on a parking lot? (Are you parking your energy, in other words?) How are the brakes? Do you have bumpers? These are important sub-symbols. Also, do you travel on freeways (is your way free?) or on narrow, bumpy roads? Do you ever misplace or lose your car? Obviously much more could be said on this subject. One further note: cars are probably more important to males.
bus (also street-car, ship, etc.)	Probably a birth symbol. It's very important to know about your birth. If you are fortunate enough to have your mother available, ask her what happened. Was it hard? easy? How long did

SYMBOL	SIGNIFICANCE AND/OR DISPOSITION
	it take? Reassure her that it is helpful to tell the truth. Often they think they have to "lie" about this "for your own good." Your dream symbols will often allude to your birth.
chairs	Possesive symbols. They hold up your rear end, don't they? We don't need furniture in a dream. Get rid of the rigid "furniture" in your life.
clothing	Unless incidental, should be avoided. It's a facade
colors	
red	Symbolizes "masculine", aggressive energy. (Remember that *all* humans are compounded of *both* masculine and feminine qualities. Capitalize on it!)
blue green	Denote feminine qualities — sensitivity, intuition, etc. Use them.
brown orange yellow gold	Possessive colors. Find out how they apply and get rid of them (They probably refer to Mama.)
purple violet	Conflict colors. Investigate!
black	If the color of an object — anxiety. If of a person, sexual, passionate; convert him/her to an ally.

SYMBOL	SIGNIFICANCE AND/OR DISPOSITION
pink	A weak red. Can you intensify it?
white	Color of authority: dependency on Mama. Assume all authority for yourself in the dream.
dirt	Guilt symbol. (See also "washing".)
disasters (earthquakes, air raids, tornadoes, etc.)	Very auspicious! They are beneficial because all the old, dependent negative parts of yourself and your world can be destroyed and a new you in a new world created. Celebrate! What are you getting rid of? What can spring up in its place? What else can you wreak havoc with that perhaps your dream neglected? After all, it's your dream.
(the) East (China, India, etc.)	A birth symbol. Beautiful! Foster it. Use it. You can birth and grow yourself in a few seconds. Do it.
England	At least for Americans (even those whose forefathers came from Italy and Eastern Europe or Germany or where-have-you) this spells Mother Country. Get it? Find out why. What does she still possess of yours? Get it back! Kitchens are also mother country. Dreams are tricky and playful — play along with them and you'll figure them out.

SYMBOL	**SIGNICICANCE AND/OR DISPOSITION**
food (plates, utensils, kitchens, etc.)	No point in eating in the dream: they are a sign of dependency, of Mama. Get rid of them.
guns	Nothing surprising here — they are sex symbols. As with our comment on cars, it's important to know the age and type. (Revolver, pistol, rifle, cannon, popgun?) Is there enough ammunition? Are you misfiring? Drawing blanks? Dreams have a lot of fun with these symbols, but it's serious fun — pay attention!
rocks (stones, mountains, etc.)	These are impervious, inmovable, and inflexible rigidities in *you*. What are they? Have a dialogue with them. Then pulverize them and level the area. Enrich the soil, then grow something on the new land.
shoes	If not incidental, they are symbols of guilt — as is dirt — which they protect you from.
steps	Indicate levels of existence or stages of growth. Confront them. Discover your progression. Or regression? Perhaps they are saying you are going over your head — or living in your head (head-tripping).
teeth	Attaching, clutching, possessive instruments. Get rid of them. (That doesn't mean you need to be toothless!)

SYMBOL	SIGNIFICANCE AND/OR DISPOSITION
train	Womb symbol. (The locomotive is Mother!) Be a conductor and check out all the cars — are they cold, hot, bumpy, rattly, suffocating? What are the tracks like? and the railroad "bed"? After you get through with the survey, blow up the train and tracks. Wipe them out. You don't need this vestigital dependency tracking and training you. (This is not a lame attempt at humor but a recognition of dream language.)
vacuum cleaner	A negative energy symbol: it collects dirt and therefore guilt. Where does the dirt come from? (see "washing")
washing	Indication of guilt — about what? Fantasize getting rid of it and eliminating the image derived from others but now a part of you that threatens you with guilt. There is a strong element of anger and resentment to guilt! Defecate it! Get something growing with the fertilizer.
washing machine	A positive symbol: you're washing the guilt away. Be sure to let the machine go through all the "cycles".
water (a body of)	Refers to your birth. Dry it up — it takes just a few seconds — and then investigate the relics, debris, and teaasures lying on the bottom. Decide what you want to do with them. Then grow a new crop on this rich soil.
(the) West	Death symbol. Highly positive! — death precedes regeneration. What is dying? Accelerate the process. Replace it with something new. Birth something — like a new you.

BACKGROUND ELEMENTS

Recurring dreams are especially significant since their message is so important it must be repeated — because the dreamer refuses to pay attention. They indicate stubborn behavior patterns preventing new growth and development.

On the other hand, any unusual dream image indicates an emerging part of yourself from which new awareness and behavior can develop.

In fact a dream is always a psycho-spiritual happening reflecting a felt need to re-order our personality-world. Morever it can become a conscious rehearsal for change if we remember that all parts of the dream are parts of ourselves in need of further integration and that by changing the role and destiny of our dream symbols in fantasy or in dream we can also change our real lives.

Dreams show us not only what we're avoiding but also what we are doing - that is, the existential background, the context, of our life, which is generally symbolized by the dream setting. Whether the day is sunny or cloudy; the place, a forest, desert or cliffside; the time, day or night; the space, tight, enclosed and compartmentalized or else open and liberated; the pace, slow and torpid or energetic and lively; the "palette," black-and-white or in color; the feeling, scary, angry, frustrating, or sad, or else happy and exhilarating; the tone, ironic, alienated, approving, or positive — all these background elements contribute to a full picture of the dreamer's world.

Another key is the way the story is told. Is the dreamer the narrator or one of the players? Is there a dream within a dream? Is this a review of the past or perhaps a portent of the future? Or else is there a sense of timelessness?

The cast of characters is also significant: is it animate, inanimate or both; varied or repetitive; solitary of multiple? (If your dreams are rarely populated by human beings, we would suggest a need for individual counseling.)

If we could confront all the factors that impinge on any specific dream to make it the unique production every dream is, we would indeed be liberated! But two factors prevent us from doing this. One is the inevitable omission and forgetting of many elements of the dream. (This tendency will of course recede as we become more aware and relaxed in our dreaming, but it will always be present.)

The other factor is the principle of urgency. of priority. It is natural to give priority to those dream elements that say the most to us. They stay in the foreground; the rest tend to dim out.

But nothing is lost. The dreams roll on. In fact, a single dream offers only one facet of the dreamer's multiple notions of himself and the world; and that is why dreams should be read in series or at least in context with past dreams, so that any one dream will not distort the variegated qualities we all possess.

The main thing is to be aware that the dream is a tool for living; in fact, that it is part of living and that through it we can find new perspectives and new possibilities in life as we become more aware of the corrective images that it offers.

Techniques for handling dreams are important of course; but even more vital is a friendly ongoing relationship with our Dream Mind. All it requires is that we develop a comraderie with it and that we trust its powers. (Actually they are *our* powers.) If we do, we will dream "to any distance in any direction" and our lives must reflect that collaboration.

Meditation:

THE CUTTING EDGE OF CONSCIOUSNESS

Just like the character in a Moliere play who was astounded to learn he had been speaking prose all his life — you've been meditating all your life. Meditation is not esoteric or mystic or even special. It is a common activity we all *must* engage in. However, it is important to understand what you have been doing so that you can do it more effectively, so that you can *consciously* employ meditation as your "viewmaster" on the path toward oneness.

One thing is certain: you don't have to go to Katmandu to do it, nor join a Buddhist order, or don a loin cloth — let alone seclude yourself in the desert for forty days of solitude or be intiated into its mysteries with LSD or the magic mushroom.

On the contrary — you have *willy-nilly* been meditating ever since childhood. Meditation is a *mode* of life. It is as Indian as curry, as Chinese as tea, as Russian as borscht — and as American as apple pie. It actually comes with the territory of being human. Meditation is seeing, it is vision. It is the seeing that results from relating the self to the world (the other). Sometimes, indeed, the self seems to merge with the other (for aren't they one?) in an experience of great meaning; but that merging — no matter how beautiful or important — must not be allowed to blind us to our daily "run-of-the-mill" seeing that is the seed bed which can nurture our memorable ahah's!, insights, and epiphanies.

Yet many *are* blinded. The monks in the Himalayas performing feats of sanctity, the gurus hibernating for months in blocks of ice, and even the thousands of Americans possessed of their secret mantras have obscured the universal nature of the meditative mode. We do not realize that the tool of consciousness which all humans fashion to see the world in relation to themselves is the cutting edge we call meditation.

Of course that cutting edge can be sharpened by practice, and by knowledge and tutelage, but the experience of meditation is a human one. In fact, it is inescapable; for without it we literally cannot survive outside the walls of a supportive mental health institution.

Actually, meditation is a *range* of levels of vision — some common, some extraordinary and exalted; yet their source is that same cutting edge. And the primary fact is we are all capable of using our meditative faculty *at any time* to discover both useful and even startling insights about ourselves.

Occasionally, vision "just" occurs — though we tend to forget our incubatory psychic activity that has ushered it into the light. For example, this happened to me several years ago.

I don't even remember what I was troubled about. All I know is that I was anguished about a conflict between two alternatives as I lay in bed, in the early morning hours, waiting to hear the morning newspaper thud on the porch as a signal to start a bleary day. I had been tossing for hours. It all seemed hopeless.

And then something happened. A voice spoke. It was mine but it was a voice I had not willed, and it broadcast from a sound booth I did not know existed. It simply said: "You seem to have a conflict." That's all. But that's all I needed. I immediately felt an ineffable calm. I *accepted* the conflict. I cried out of relief and the conflict — once it was accepted — soon vanished..

That was the meditative Voice, that was the Self that *all* of us can contact, whether we believe we're meditators or not. But — once again — our Voices are occasional happenings in the main meditative performance we all enact. Not that they're not important — even significant and crucial; yet they still can only be seen in concert with our regular meditative stance. However, they are a valuable resource, and so it would be useful if we could meet *our* Overseeing Self in this first meditative exercise:

1.   It would be helpful to sit straight (in a chair or not).

2.   Close your eyes and expel the stale air in the lungs 4 times. (Notice you need not worry about inhaling — this happens naturally and deeply if *all* the stale air is pushed out.)

3. Watch yourself breathe for 3 minutes. (Notice how the breathing begins to relax and flow — while it deepens.)

4. Now watch your thoughts for 5 minutes. (We'll discuss "thoughts" later on; right now just watch them.) By watching, we mean: observing, not holding on to them, treating them like a movie projectionist. Do this longer than 5 minutes if you do find yourself holding on to any of them.

5. Now the "screen" is probably empty. (If it isn't that's all right too: it's a most human condition.) Review with attentive *objectivity* three conflicts in *your* life. Put 3 questions about each conflict: (a) What is it exactly? (No pondering. The first "guess" will almost undoubtedly be right!); (b) Must I hold on to it? (If the answer is Yes, that's O.K.); (c) How can I get rid of it if I don't want it anymore?

DISCUSSION

It is amazing how much underbrush can be cleared away with this simple exercise. We often don't realize how dead many "conflicts" are. If they are dead, how can you resolve them? (By telling someone you feel differently now? By simply acting toward a person or a problem as if the conflict were no longer there? By just letting go? How else?)

For those conflicts you must for now hold on to, just put one question about each: Could I make some headway toward resolving this if I were to discharge some painful emotions that are now stopping me? (If the answer is even a partial yes, see Chapter 2 for further assistance.)

When obstacles in your life take the form of problems that cannot be reduced to either-or conflicts, it is difficult to attack them. In such cases, the following exercise often helps amazingly to clarify their personal significance. With a problem in mind . . .

1. Repeat the first 3 directions of the first exercise until you feel at ease.

2. Now look at your problem with attentive objectivity. (Imagine that it belongs to a friend and not to you: you are interested surely but not *involved.*)

3. Then ask yourself: "What kind of person would attract this problem?" (Or: "Whom does this tempt?"; "Whom does this pain?", etc.)

4. Pause for mental quiet. Resume the placid breathing if necessary.

5. Repeat the questions in No. 3 until the answer seems "right." It shouldn't take long. (After all, who knows you better than your Self!)

DISCUSSION

No doubt you will once again be amazed at the objectivity, the total awareness, of the Self. You will discover the longer you consciously meditate that the Self does not identify with the body, the intellect, or the feelings and emotions but seems to possess a Martian objectivity. Glory in it. Cherish it. It can save your life!

Caution: Perhaps the Self will tell you that the child in you that your father rarely loved when you were young feels abandoned or that the fearful you was once afraid that your mother wouldn't survive, or that the jealous you is *also* unfaithful — regardless ....Just remember you have two possibilities: (a) You may decide that the feelings of abandonment, fear, jealousy, etc., are dead and that you can say goodby to them. Or, (b) you may realize the potency of these feelings even though they might have been generated years ago and decide you want to work through them. We urge: By all means do! Suppressed feelings do not leave until they're discharged. (see Chapter 2 for assistance.)

One purpose of these exercises is to share meditation with the mystics, gurus, and the saints (and this is not said disrespectfully) so that *all of us* can begin to see how fundamental it is to our existence. For example, the phrase "peak experience" is bandied around, as if only special people have them — preferably with halos, or at least special robes. But we all have peak experiences, they blossom from *our* meditative capacities — they are simply accurate seeings that "happen" when we suddenly look just right at the world. It is important to be aware of this resource too, for our awareness is the general field in which meditation is cultivated. That is why it would be useful to recover this aspect of our history also in the following exercise:

1. Repeat the first 3 directions of the first exercise until you feel at ease, hopefully placid.

2. Look at your total life with attentive objectivity.

3. Recall some "peak experiences" you had with nature. Do this (and the other categories to be reviewed) chronologically. Perhaps the experience was "dramatic" (like a mountain climb); or suprising (like the bird who stared at you while you stared at it); or shocking (like an animal killing its prey); or opening (like a sunset); or? . . .

4. Ask a friend (peer counselor, lover, colleague, etc.) if possible to follow the above steps also.

5. Then take turns listening to each other (or tell them to yourself). Relive these precious experiences. Take your time. If feelings well up, allow them to "happen."

6. Now review peak experiences in games, dance, athletics, war, etc. Share them, if possible, as in Step 5.

7. Follow the same procedures with the categories of *work* and *people*. (Take your time. All of these are broad and rich categories to be mined with expectant zeal.)

DISCUSSION

How has the inclusion of peak experiences changed your notion of meditation? Can you come to some conclusions about *your way* of "connecting" with these experiences? (This is an important consideration.) How challenging would integrating this way into your life pattern be? Are some changes possible now? Can you consider the possibility that some peaks would be normal occurrences if you could remove the blocks that usually obscure them? How far are you willing to go? Can you set some goals now? Return to this discussion after you finish this chapter — and the book; it could be rewarding . . .

Review

It would be good to survey where we have gone thus far. First we have stated that meditation is a mode of life common to us all. Then we defined meditation as that characteristic perceptual stance each of us takes as we consciously relate to our environment. Lastly, we showed that all of us possess not only the general skill of meditation but also some of its special capabilities that can shed light on the deepest recesses of our personality.

Three questions remain: Where did meditation come from? how did it evolve? Then: how can we sharpen its cutting edge so that we can *consciously* use it as a basic tool in the process of living and being? And finally — how does meditation as a special act (with prescribed postures, mantras, schedules, and religious-philosophical attitudes) fit into our general conception?

History

Obviously the meditative faculty was not discovered like electricity or gravity. No one flew a kite or watched an apple fall. It evolved. But one "event" had to precede it: humankind had to "decide" that they were not only a part of nature, like the rest of the animal kigdom, but could change and control it as well — and this "decision" turned out to be the first and most radical of all human revolutions. In fact, we are still feeling its reverberations, today perhaps more sharply than ever.

For there was both gain and loss with this "new" undertaking. With control over nature our ancestors evolved the power of consciousness — the power to imagine, to analyze, to plan, to create, and to change. But there was a price to pay too: a separation *from* nature, so that humans could now feel fearful, alone, and naked (the Garden of Eden) with their new virtuosity... And so the fear of a mysterious — if not malevolent — universe outside the Garden often deflected thought into delusion, daydream, and mental "chatter." Freedom came with a price as it always does...

But human beings began to realize that their prized possession — thought, consciousness — could control that chatter through the process of *thinking about thinking*, of being aware *of their thinking*, or being aware of the way they perceived reality, of being aware of the continual discrepancies between the objective reality they already partially understood and the figments and confusions their minds created.

Moreover, they eventually began to realize that this thinking about thinking — this supervision of our mental productions which we call meditation — could not only bring harmony to the troubled mind but also — and therefore — a *reunion* with nature, a re-entry into the Garden that we and our ancestors have always dreamt about.

Then why is it that the re-entry has taken so long, that we're still outside the gates of Eden? Since we have the "technology," why has the dream been deferred?

The main reason is human oppression which has subjected the mass of humankind throughout most of history to a division of labor that has prevented them from reclaiming their full powers — while the few who *consciously* employed meditation for a new reconciliation with nature generally used it, in part, as a means of insulating themselves from the conflicts and alienations of the society. But the question is — can such meditators truly reconcile with nature while separated from the mass of humanity? We think not.

Since insulation was a traditional attitude in the Far East, the main source of our knowledge about meditational disciplines, it is no wonder that in the West meditation still retains its occult aura — which is indeed unfortunate, for *our* division of labor need exclude few from its practice. Especially will it exclude few if we conceive of meditation as a mode of life — and not a special activity requiring assigned periods of the day for its practice. Nor does this mean we depreciate the value of meditation as a special act: we only suggest the special act be seen in context with our main meditative practice *in life itself.*

Stemming from human oppression* comes another key reason for the deferral of the dream: the long-belated discovery that discharge of distress (and suppressed) feelings can liberate human beings to recover their innate powers of rationality for making this world a more attractive abode.

But *together* discharge and meditation can perform as powerful engines for human growth and change especially since they are *reciprocally* beneficial: for discharge opens new vistas for meditation while meditation discovers new conflicts to discharge, so that we can envision ever-broader and deeper understandings of our selves and the universe.

Using Meditation

Now we face the question, How do we sharpen the cutting edge so that meditation serves discharge — and discharge, meditation?

By returning — as always when we need to feel bedrock — to our Fundamental Belief that human beings are unique, beautiful, loving, creative, intelligent, and zestful creatures. Even ourselves! And when they're not feeling or acting that belief — then distress is conflicting their feelings, crippling their behavior, and distorting their vision.

But how, since distress is well-nigh universal, can we — regardless — develop a creative cutting edge to our meditation? By courageously and resolutely cleaving to that Belief even though our feelings scream that it can't be done, that it's all a myth, that people are evil and the world is rotten. Often you will need to take that Belief on faith alone when the world "out there" is dim and your hurt feelings are running like a torrent — but take the Belief anyway, hold onto it, cleave to it, and it will see you through! For "it" *is* you — you the diamond needing only polish to glisten.

---

*See page 25, Chapter 1

So how do you work then? You take a stand *for* the Belief, you take a direction *toward* the Belief, and you formulate a "statement" *out of* that Belief which will incorporate a positive image of yourself so that you can now see the world and yourself with the cutting edge of that positive thrust.

First, a "routine" example that seems simplistic but yet can deftly undercut a gibbering invalidating pattern: If you walk into a room feeling inferior to those you haven't met and knowing surely you won't be liked, just say to yourself, "I am intelligent and everyone loves me!" If you say it knowing truly that you are of course intelligent — which indeed you are — and that those in the room are loving — which indeed all humans are — then you will be amazed at the efficacy of this "simple" statement. You will quickly discover that what is simple is not necessarily simplistic!

A more personal example: Just a few mornings before I wrote this I felt defeatist and despondent as I opened my eyes to face the day. Nor was it easy to recognize that my feelings were unrealistic — for my deepest distress lies in feelings of hopelessness. However, I did finally recognize my upset and so I asked myself (with the Belief in mind): "What do I need to say to confront my distress?" The answer came back quickly as an echo: "It's a good life!" This meant for me that I was O.K. and the world was too — and that made sense surely, now that my distressed feelings had subsided (after causing some discharge).

So I had a direction, I had an edge, and I took that edge and I applied it to my life that day. I tried to *feel* that total O.K.-ness as I navigated on my pathways in the world that day. I tried to *see* the world with that total O.K.-ness as I navigated on my pathways in the world that day. I tried to *be* that total O.K.-ness as I navigated on my pathways in the world that day . . . I was largely successful. I had enormous energy and I was delighted with myself.

This was meditation. It was meditation in action. Of course some of the notions I "projected" that day on the screen of my mind were not in accord with my direction; so I noticed them with attentive objectivity, then adjusted slightly toward the direction once again, and proceeded in the O.K.-ness. That's all that was needed — just a slight correction.

Sometimes more is needed — including a firm resolve to hold the direction even though there is a hard counter-pull. Very often you will discharge after such a successful resolve; or else you might need to put a check on an inappropriate flow of feelings until you can recount the experience to a friend or your own self-counselor at the first opportunity. But one thing must be clear: this is not Norman Vincent Peale's "power of positive thinking," for his rigid stances are not recommended.

The alternatives are not "positive thinking" — or else the skids. Progress through discharge and meditation are certain. You can always assume that you are doing the best you can and that if there are slips and falls they must be caused by distress you need to look at. And you can and you will . . . Meanwhile the picture of the Belief remains, the picture of yourself as its living embodiment remains; and so there is no conflict, and thus the way to oneness is unimpeded and free. Basically, it is free because at their core the Belief describes *all human beings**. With the staff of that Belief in your hand, therefore, the way is clear, though the struggle may be arduous.

I have *general* directions also for returning my ship to its course. Two of my favorites, likewise, confront feelings of hopelessness. One is "simply" a YES . . . Yet how unsimple it is to feel that YES! to sense it in my fiber, to radiate it — but mainly to accept it.For it is already there when I uncover it under the dourness...and the hurts laid down.

The other direction says much the same thing, but in a slightly different way. It's "just" a smile. But once again: how hard to smile in your toes, to twinkle in your knees, to grin with your breath, to enjoy with your blood, and to laugh in your heart! *That* is a fine meditation! You will truly learn much about yourself as you watch your negative mental "static" sputter through that one.

All of us of course — perhaps with the help of a friend, guide, or self-counselor — must fashion directions for ourselves, for only we know how to reach the soul while dealing with relevant limitations. We can make adjustments as we go along. Each day might need finer calibration — or else a new channel. The art of maintaining the edge is the sophistication of meditation.

---

*unless they have been physically damaged in a special way.

Now it might be good to review the recent thread of our discussion — especially for readers who are meditating in more conventional ways. We want to say to you: if those ways are helpful, carry on, don't change. But perhaps even though your particular techniques won't alter, your understanding of the *relationship* between meditation and life activity might subtly affect the whole. We earnestly hope so.

In any case for us — and for the hundreds we've observed use the Cutting Edge Technique — it is vastly helpful to see reality not only with the clarity of vision we can currently develop (given the status of our individual distress) but also with the Fundamental Belief that we can by nature transcend that clarity since we are by nature unique, beautiful, loving, creative, intelligent, and zestful beings.

For in our experience we have often observed *our* seeing skewed by *our* distress. Furthermore, we have observed many long-term traditional meditators who have locked themselves in to deep seated distress patterns *through* their meditative pratice — and this is said with sincere understanding.

The fact is that distress patterns are stubborn, rigid *mechanisms* that seem perfectly natural to their owner although they delude us into seeing through our glass darkly. But things are never simple. Traditional meditation is often accompanied by discharge and therefore new insights and therefore more lucid meditation and therefore additional discharge. We are aware that the Cutting Edge Technique has no monopoly on this reciprocal process.

Our main point is that positive direction can deepen the cutting edge and thus speed up personal regeneration. Moreover, it can help us avoid the danger of accomodating not only to personal limitations but to environmental disfunctions as well. Oneness cannot be achieved at the price of others just as liberation for others cannot be reached with the enslavement of one. Meditation is a pratice that must include the wide world, for the individual is a reflection of that world and no degree of isolation can cut that inner relationship.

To put it another way: just as thinking about thinking (which is essentially what meditation is) can steer us around many pitfalls, so thinking about thinking about thinking can even further illuminate and deepen the meditative process. For the Cutting Edge is that additional thinking factor, it is that additional fulcrum, that additional center we can employ to join with our true selves and our brothers and sisters to create a greener land and a brighter people.

Essentially, we differ with traditional meditative pratice on only one theoretical point. Traditionalists claim that meditation needs to deal with our mental static — our own uncontrolled inner computers — to achieve oneness. We agree; but we believe one step has been left out. We are convinced that reactive feelings energize mental static so that meditative practice cannot be divorced from sound emotional practice — in fact they must dovetail in mutual support — if we are to arrive at wholeness.

With that mutual support we then agree that seeing is meditation and truly seeing is love and seeing truly brings beauty and delight.

Finding Your Guide

I have my own private spiritual guide. I call on him regularly. He is so close that I cannot reveal his name.

But the process of finding one for yourself I do want to reveal; for I know that for you — as well as me — there are days of conflict, of spiritual turmoil, emotional crisis, when words of wisdom — or perhaps simply just a reassuring smile — can pacify your troubled waters and give you courage to go on. Your Guide, actually, can prevail for you on a day-to-day basis.

But I'm already in deep water! I've used the word *spiritual* as if we have a common dictionary. But perhaps we can compile one. Let's see . . .

But first — I am not referring to any specific religious figure or practice. Nor is a belief in the divine a requirement. Rather, I am referring to that dimension in all of us which glows at a smiling child, expands at certain sounds of music, gleams with pride for family or nation or humanity, responds to needs of unseen multitudes, and opens in unselfish love for another; or perhaps that dimension which stands exposed before a turbulent sea, a magnificent animal, a dimly shrouded peak, or a delicate flower; or which truly sees another, intuitively, can tell what is going on "instinctively," and is there when a crisis is dire and hope seems gone; there, just a breath away, in a heartbeat revealed.

Does that explain what *spiritual* means? Of course not! And yet, perhaps, it can take you within its vicinity if you will use these words as road signs indicating intersecting *directions* so that the point at which they cross cold be your spiritual dimension even though I have not identified it like Boston or Los Angeles or Des Moines.

Another difficulty with navigating in spiritual waters is that many people will acknowledge spiritual qualities in others, but not in themselves. Who? — me!?

Yes, you . . .all of us. We are all amalgams compounded in part of spirit. But that is a false statement too. Spirit is not a distinct substance separate from matter but rather a quality of the whole, a way of being of the whole, a function of the whole human being. In part, words are responsible for the confusion for we have none that can adequately describe the subtleties of our human potential.

But, once again, so many people are removed from this aspect of their nature They do not realize how accidental is the formation of our "character" — how our history, our parents, our environment "choose" some *few special qualities* in us, of all our myriad possibilities, that *conveniently fit our early life situation.* And so we freeze in that mold!

So few of us understand that we would need a thousand lifetimes to discover the potential of our possibilities in all their combinations! Most of us bank our fires low, not realizing we are all one: all compounded of the same essence, all searching (if unawarely) for self-realization. We are capable not only of discovering a personal Guide but of creating a series of them throughout a lifetime to nurture our evolving growth. (I have had but three, since I started late.) My present one is an inner light, a solace, a wisdom-bearer, a helpmate, a friend.

And yours? How would you make contact with your Source, your Guide? First, believe that you can! At the least allow the *possibility* to lurk and then grow somewhere inside of you. Treat it like a guest and the newcomer will soon feel at home in the regions of your psyche where he/she needs to preside. At the least, play "as if," — that will probably be enough — because I am convinced, whatever you want to call it, however you want to interpret it or explain it, that you do have an inner intelligence that can radiate to the perimeter of your being in times of need. It's a question of *recognizing* its presence.

How do you discover your guide? First, let's test where your inclinations lead. We need to feed your unconscious with personal data (like a dating bureau) so that your "computer" will do its work efficiently in order to link up with your Mate. Think about the following questions. Let the answers percolate and nourish the subsoil. Take your time with this questionnaire. Add questions of your own: you know best how to contact your essence.

A Spiritual Inventory

1. Would your guide be male or female? Of what age? Color? Nationality? Religion? Race?
2. In what country would your guide appear?
3. Under what conditions would you expect to find him/her? Under stress? In a contemplative mood? While dreaming? In nature? In church? Meditating?.
4. Would your guide be an actual person or, rather, a composite of valuable qualities? Or perhaps a symbol? a light? a color? a sound? a touch?
5. In what setting are you most creative?
6. Has an experience in nature awakened your spiritual dimension?
7. Has a work of art (including a song, book, movie, or play) opened up unexpectedly your inner horizons?
8. Is your spirituality related to contributing to mankind. — like Albert Schweitzer or Martin Luther King?
9. Do you see science including a spiritual vision? If so, what scientist do you feel akin to?
10. Have you ever experienced remarkable spirituality in a "simple," "ordinary" person?
11. Is there a race or people (perhaps of a particular historical period) who possess an admirable spiritual sense? Is there a figure. — real or symbolic — who represents this group for you?
12. Who is the most altruistic person in your experience? In history? In your *experienced* religious life?
13. Who was the most spiritually wise person you've known?

14.   When were you most spiritually open? Was there a figure whom you associated your spirituality with?

15.   Do you recall an experience that opened up a new realm of thinking or feeling for you — like a revelation?

16.   Recall the times when your heart "opened." How did it happen?

17.   Is there a meaningful spiritual figure who inhabits your inner space?

18.   What is the most nourishingly beautiful experience you cherish?

Setting The Stage

Let some time intervene between the inventory and what we shall do next — perhaps a whole day or longer, for a gestation period. Before going to sleep it would be helpful to think about how your spirituality functions. Review the data the inventory revealed. Make it available to your dream mind. Ask your dream mind to help you see your Guide within. If you are serious, it will! (Keep a notebook and pen handy by your beside to write down your dream.)

Now we can proceed to the next stage of our search. For this you need to recall and envision your Zone of Peace — an actual place in the geography of your life where you can go for calm and solace. It is such a natural place for you to be you that it almost seems a mirror of you, a region of ease within you. But it exists!

It is a real place, a place in the real world where you have felt totally at ease, where — when you approach its environs — a sigh will surprisingly release, as if to say, "I am home."

Find *your* Zone. Mine is the ocean, a particular beach really. I know what the gulls look like there and the shore birds with their razor beaks; the lagoon and the farther headlands and the beach homes; the stones, a jellyfish, a sand dollar; a sail, the smoke from a distant ship; the aroma of the sea, its perennial pounding, the garrulous air filled with inspiriting energy — this and so much more that must be wordless in my Zone of Peace to which I return to find my Guide...

What is your Zone like? Reflect upon it with eyes closed now. You know it. Let it come to you. Be a receptive screen upon which the images from your zone can congregate and coalesce to become a place to retreat to when you need a message that can help you steer through rough waters. Take your time and then we'll proceed . . .

The Practice

Now let's sink into ourselves. With eyes closed, do some deep breathing: first fill the belly, the chest, the shoulders (make them rise); then let it all out, expel all the air; sigh it all out as if you were giving it all up. Make a noise, use your voice box, feel the marvelous giving-in (the surrender to your Self).

And then again — the breathing, the letting-go. Do this for three minutes. Sink . . .into the Self.

Now count slowly from 12 to 1 (this should take approximately one minute), relaxing the head, the eyes, the neck, the shoulders, the back, the chest, solar plexus, genital area, legs and feet.

Say to yourself: "I am now at a deeper level of my being."

Then count again — from 10 to 1 — this time feeling yourself sink into those dry recesses, those arid places that are so rarely filled in the anxious hurly-burly of our lives. Feel your juices fill the places that have been dry so long.

Say to yourself: "I am now at the deepest level of my being."

Feel the calm, the repose. Feel the Self unencumbered.

Now let the Self inhabit the Zone of Peace that you designed for your repose. Still with eyes closed, look at all its features with natural delight. Survey them in a particular order and maintain this order whenever you return to your Zone. See how satisfying they are, how calming they are, how harmonious for your Guide to preside over. Feel sure that your Guide *can* preside over this scene: after all it was to *your inner powers* that it first appealed to!

Now begin to look around, still with eyes closed. Where would your Guide appear? Look there assuredly. Allow your Guide space to manifest — don't push, don't demand. Your Guide is there — be confident of that.

When you finally meet, greet your Guide, have a dialogue. Ask for a blessing, a word, a caution, a message of love. They will be forthcoming — and you will have found a North Star that you can always take your bearings from.

There is one cautionary note to be added at this point: be patient. Finding your appointed Guide can be a process lasting a few days or even a few weeks. But in all probability your Guide will appear in your first "invocation."

Remember that its form and identity could change through time as your Self adjusts and correlates its needs in your expanding life. *But do not reveal the form and identity to anyone.* That would be squandering spiritual capital!

Eventually — or so it has happened to me — a long-term partnership will develop.

Your Guide awaits. Be sure of it. Have a beautiful life together!

KEEPING THE POWER

When we are one, the spirit dances

Cook Your Rice

Would you go on a trip if you didn't know what it is you're going to see? Even if at the very end there might be gaps and mysteries? Your life is like that of course (and so is mine) — but this is a chapter in a book and at least here you wold expect clarity and coherence. But sometimes coherence can only come at the very end of a trip — and even then be unspoken! And the clarity might come and go like reflections mirrored on water.

In fact if you become too sure of what I mean, I could very well have failed. For some learnings grow organically, we grope for them: they *emerge*, like ever clearer photographs, as we learn to focus better.

However when they're *interior* visions we need snapshots from many angles and perspectives and levels so that the picture that does emerge will at least point to the reality. But perhaps I fear the very thing I want to talk about — success. Success is just the tip of the iceberg, but that is where we must start.

But stop! I must adjust the camera again. (Be patient, we will begin soon. You will just have to believe for a little while longer that Cooking Rice *is* a delicate project.) I do not *necessarily* mean success but, at least initially, the *feeling* of success, the anticipation of success. We can start there.

Since I'm a writer, I think of an example that all writers must have experienced: the surrendering of a fruitful idea to write about as a consequence of talking about it to one's friends. It is such a temptation! They are intrigued, they are mystified; they are delighted; and one wants so much to share the joy of creation, the joy of anticipation, the joy of working through the myriad problems one faces that the very seeds of creation are spilled in masturbatory verbalization... And so all is lost, surrendered, given up.

Serious writers learn to *cook their rice*: not to release the power that is incubating inside them but to nurture it, protect it, conceal it (like an embryo) until it is ready for birth. Then it is time enough to talk and expand and celebrate the *doing,* the creation.

Moreover one can lose creative power in internal dialogue just as surely — and more commonly. Writers can regale *themselves* with their prowess, all they need is an audience of one to hear about their daring craftsmanship and their remarkable persistence in producing — the inevitable miscarriage.

It is indeed a profound problem. Talk (both inner and outer) is a threat to the "rice." It is especially a critical problem in a society like ours that is based on merchandising both people and products (sometimes they're indistinguishable!). For the merchandising is largely based on talk and even the talker can be taken in by his own spiel. (Ask any salesman.)

A remarkable example of this delusion takes place in Arthur Miller's play, "Death of a Salesman." It is a play about Willy Loman, who was one of the old-time salesmen who opened up new territories for their companies, who developed "connections" and relationships to push their products, who in truth created a viable world — but yet one that was mainly based on webs of words.

So it was that when the real world beyond the words changed, the salesmen were lost. They just hadn't noticed how television, radio, and the newspaper more efficiently sold their products, and at less cost. Willy could not understand what had happened. Each sale had buttressed his dream, his self-image, and now the selling days were over and he "therefore" was through too. His "rice" had been based on words.

As had been that of his sons. Willy had expected that his son Biff would become a great success because he was a star football player in high school — and the words that surrounded him *were* glowing. Biff believed those words too so that he never discovered his *inner* substance.

He didn't study, he failed in school; the promised college scholarships no longer dangled before his eyes, and so his ego collapsed. The world of words had betrayed him. But the playwright purposely contrasts Willy and Biff with Charley (a loyal friend of

Willy's) and Bernard, his son. Charley is skeptical, even cynical, of the huckstering world, and Bernard at the beginning is an awkward adolescent with no campus glamor, but he does possess a curiosity about the world and himself that permits him to build on inner strengths.

Later Bernard becomes a lawyer and we meet him and Willy in Charley's office. Bernard is there to say goodby to his father before leaving for Washington.

To Willy's question about what he's going to do he merely says, "oh, just a case I've got there, Willy."

And then Charley comes in, puts his arm around his son, and says to Willy, "How do you like this kid? Gonna argue a case in front of the Supreme Court."

Willy is shocked: "No! The Supreme Court!"

After Bernard leaves, Willy says, "The Supreme Court! And he didn't even mention it!"

Charley replies, "He don't have to — he's gonna do it."

Even after a "victory" talk can be dangerous. How many love *affairs* and permanent relationships too are stillborn because sexual consummation is confused with oneness. — because the energy from the consummation is translated into ego-inflating illusions that both blind the individual and waste energy. Just when an I-thou relationship could "take off," self-congratulatory (inner) talk blinds one from the other, and so dries and scatters the bitter rice.

The fable of the tortoise and the hare also concerns the same danger: that dread point when "success" is so close that the preening ego splits off from the self on a self-congratulatory detour. The hare had plenty of time to gloat, to cavort, to snooze; but he lost the race because he did not tend the rice. The tortoise did. Never was there a clevage in its mind between the doing and the being. The tortoise and the race were one. In fact, winning was beside the point. The race simply had to be run just as a tortoise must run it. The "victory" was someone else's headline.

Cooking your rice is a subtle concept. One of its subtleties is that ends are but new beginnings — and who knows the "proper" label, if we must have labels? The only thing we do know — or can know — is the permanence of change, but that's sometimes hard to hold on to. Well do I know it!...

I once went through the process of primal therapy. It was rich and rewarding. It was the first time I experienced the suppressed feelings that I had carried around like a packhorse for fifty years. I learned to cry and to laugh, to hate and to love; and then when blockages crashed all around me, thoughts blossomed. I was in seventh heaven, I had climbed Everest, I had arrived. I even got The Key: just a few days before the three-week intensive was over my therapist told me I could leave my enforced isolation and go out into the world again.

I had practically *graduated!* (I didn't ask myself from what.) I would celebrate! — which meant to me: *at least* eat a good meal . . .

I was near Sausalito at the time — a delightfully invigorating (though touristy) little town just the other side of San Francisco Bay. I would go there, of course, promenade the streets, window-shop disdainfully (for I now had everything), and then feast appropriately.

But alas! — it was a Monday and the good restaurants were closed. How awful! How insufferably awful! I raged at this brusing blow. But I recovered a semblance of composure. I wold transcend the disappointment and eat anywhere: after all food was food. I thought I had achieved an Olympian calm.

I chose a perfectly decent place that was both bar and restaurant and ordered a meal, which consisted of soup, salad, and a main dish of sauteed chicken. What could be bad about that? I reassuringly asked myself.

But blows kept coming. The soup was canned — chicken, I recall. The salad, tasteless herbage. However, the main dish was still ahead . . .

And here it was. It was chicken all right — that had been steamed and then lightly fried to simulate the sauteed effect. I was crushed, but I finished it solemnly, like a sick philosopher. What could I do now? I felt stuck.

And then it happened — one of the most vivid and dramatic moments of my life . . .

I suddenly saw in my mind's eye a bruising, burly, red-haired terror of a man who looked at me straight in the eye, demanding (while relishing my helplessness): "So you deny you called me a liar!"

Immediately I knew I was trapped. If I didn't deny it, *I* would be the liar. If I did, *he* would. Either way was disaster. I was scared. It was a classic double-bind. And then the hallucination vanished (it was all just a matter of seconds). I sat there like a stone and then I began to think: how accurately the vision had enacted what I had done to *my self*. *I* had double-bound myself. I had been on a no-win path. I decided to go back to my temporary home and contemplate.

Many years have passed; yet I often think of that ruddy brute, perhaps because my expectations at times still overrun my sense of reality so that the rice is burned, instead of cooked kernel by kernel. We do not graduate from change. We become . . .

Change is "simply" a by-product of the becoming. The becoming is the fundamental process that drives all reality. Energy, enthusaism, creativity, the spark, the living Word are inherent in our entire universe. They form the substrate,the ground,of our very being: is it any wonder that we sometimes feel the ground move, the energy rise, enthusiasm peak?

But if we do not realize that this Universal Pulse is an *impersonal* force that is always there for us if we but hook into it through a process of letting go, *then* we see change as purely personal achievement — and thus an ego trip that can waylay us at any step, as it did me in Sausalito.

The irony is that the very impulse to own the ground of being cuts it off (much as external/internal talk does), for it is not ours to possess. On the contrary: the second we think we own it — we lose it!

I must tell another personal story now, for,as I said at the beginning, we are dealing with a theme that must be sneaked up on — much like the naturalist in the wilderness who knows that it is not *quite* wilderness any longer since *he* is there!

This happened at Esalen, the famed "growth center" at Big Sur, California. It was one of those memorable days when I felt hooked-in to the Universal Pulse. The air was redolent with both sun and ocean, invigorating yet warming — harmoniously zestful!

And I just had a massage from a beautiful woman. It was far more than a massage: it was an opening up, a revelation of my physical, emotional, and spiritual nature. I cried long and also laughed with a person whose name I long ago forgot; but all else is as fresh as the kelp and the sea otters that bob in the water below the high cliffs of this wondrous place.

Before that I had sat in the baths that overlook the ocean and are fed by a miraculous hot spring that the Indians had long venerated. I had sat in the water, then sunned, and sat again, until I was filled; then the massage. After, I walked.

I walked along a path because I wanted to walk. I was going nowhere — or everywhere. I was feeling only that I was walking, and simultaneously that *everything* was walking...

So was a cat — who was ambling the other way, toward me. He was black. I like black cats. I saw him. In the seeing I must have included him in my world. Who knows?

But this I do know: he jumped on me! On my shoulder. I was not frightened. I kept walking, perhaps about twenty yards, as if — that's the way it was, there happened to be a cat on my shoulder, why not?

And then my awareness changed to a consciousness of distinctions. I became *proud* of the cat. I tried to "own" him. And of course he did what cats always do when they feel that owning — they leave! He jumped. That's the whole story . . .

Yet that cat too I shall never forget — both *our* walking and his jumping: there's a lesson in both . . .

Why did he jump off? Because I had cut our *common* connection with the Universal Pulse. My ego had betrayed me. I do not berate myself for it but, frankly, marvel that it happened at all; for I know it's no one's fault that we rarely feel the Pulse. When we do, it's frightening.

After all, we live in a world of commodities, of merchandising: a world that processes objects and humans alike so that they'll be different enough to be distinguishable and yet similar enough to be definable in terms of price or some other success-failure rating.

And yet we are unqiue! Is it any wonder we cannot enjoy our rice but become more involved in the owning and packaging? We become anesthetized to the Power so that if, miraculously, it does go ON we feel we are on Stage Center with a hundred spotlights probing for our next move — and we had better not be found wanting!

So it is that we become inured to outer and inner failure since only a few of us become "stars" or "leading personalities." Soon we believe we would be counted frauds if only "they" knew, and we develop failure patterns that will fight to the death not only the occasional "rush" of energy but the more dangerous assumption that our very makeup is endowed with creativity, enthusiasm, and elegance.

To the extent that these patterns win out we become involved in depression — a process that literally presses down — and out — the natural exuberance of the human being, the natural rice that is our very essence. Failure patterns can depress the excitement of living by misusing numerous "weapons" that can be essential and even beautiful — such as food, drink, sex, relaxation, entertainment. Or they can use sophisticated specifics that rarely "fail" — alcohol, drugs, gambling.

There are so many other ways of turning off the rice, but a catalogue is not the point — you will know what your way is, and how to avoid it. Also there are many ways of seemingly *turning on* in order to turn off our Amazing Current.

We mentioned one. It is probably the most important: talking. Takling to others, to oneself. It can be a way of acting out rather than acting; of appearing, rather than being. Like an "exhibition". We can also "exhibit" with clothes, with mannerisms, with hyperactivity, with "gaiety", with "personality". Once again, you will know what your way is and how to avoid it.

Since we are after all energy systems connected with an Energy System that powers all life on this planet, we are not arguing for exclusivity, for a withholding of the joy we feel from others. On the contrary! We want authentic sharing; but that can only come about after we first experience the rice.

Sharing then becomes a form of radiation rather than an attempt to allay anxiety. Sharing becomes the vibrations we play as we live: the celebration of an experience rather than its anticipation.

Cooking your rice is investing in psychic capital rather than in emotive publicity. It is the development of a center, a foundation, a way of being.

If you are in any doubt about how to handle the joy of living, write a poem, paint a picture, give someone love — or meditate or, perhaps most appropriately, experience through self-appreciation how natural and logical it is that that this joy has come to you: how deserved it truly is.

Cook your rice, my friends! It is important that you do, for if you do it adds to the store for us all. We shall attempt to cook ours.

And good luck to us all!

Harvesting The Work

The "Journey" is over but *our* journey (yours and ours) continues. The book we write each day continues. The daily life we live each day is our book of health; and we create our health each day.

But sometimes it's a lonely job — creating health. Sometimes we want to chuck everything when we hurt — and gorge on food, get high on drugs, or hurt someone we love (including ourselves). And that's when we *have to* reach out to others for help. And if we can, that's when *we need* to help — for helping is even more healing than getting.

The main truth is: we are all sojourners on this planet: we all falter, but we can rise to help; we all feel the pull of past conditioning, but all of us can head toward the future too, breaking the bonds. The main truth is: we are all — everyone of us — doing the best we can. If we could do better, we would be! It is this profoundly simple idea that that can buoy our spirits as we daily create our health.

For it is not health programs and regimens that are important in the final analysis but that spark of life we generate in our daily life. It is the spark of creativity that we all possess; it is the awesome reservoir of intelligence that we all harbor; it is the deep potential for love that we all own — which can create our daily health. And we can all do it, everyone of us: we deeply know that.

We simply don't need old dead *stuff* to drag us down. The past has passed. Let's not look back. We can shatter the shibboleths of racism and sexism and any other-ism that degrades human beings in order to journey together — all of us!

Proclaiming our humanity is really the business of health! Let's be human in the way we eat, feel, love, and create.

And let's do it together!

Walk With Us

Walk with us as we move
Across the bridge
From the old to the new
Breaking out
Toward the oneness with
All life — and with you

Walk with us as we move
In our search
Let's walk
Dance
Create
A new world together

Together let us decipher the code
Of pain and fear
To reveal the light
In our hearts
Let us journey down
The real roads we walk on

Let us scourge
The shadows in our soul
The fear in the flesh
To find the harmony
Of our oneness
On our journey

Let us reach out
For one another
Loving each other and ourselves
Rejoicing in the earth
In the grace of peace
In the light of love

And as we journey together
Let us never forget
We have already arrived
We are already there
On our walk together
To find our beginnings.